health
promotion
strategies and methods

health
promotion
strategies and methods

third edition

Garry Egger MPH PhD M.A.P.S.
Director, Centre for Health Promotion
and Research, Sydney, NSW
Professor of Health and Human Sciences,
Southern Cross University, Lismore, NSW
Adjunct Professor of Exercise and Nutrition,
Deakin University, Melbourne, Vic
and University of South Australia, Adelaide, SA

Ross Spark MSc PhD
James Cook University, Cairns, Qld

Rob Donovan PhD
Professor of Behavioural Research,
Curtin University, Perth, WA

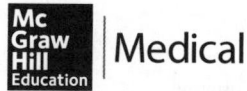

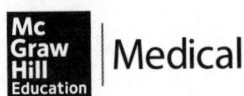
Medical

First edition 1990
Revised 1999
Reprinted 2002
Second edition 2005
Reprinted 2005, 2009
Third edition 2013

National Library of Australia Cataloguing-in-Publication data:

Author: Egger, Garry.
Title: Health promotion strategies and methods/Garry Egger
ISBN: 9781743071830 (paperback)
Notes: Includes index.
Previous edition: 2005
Subjects: Health education.
          Health promotion.
Dewey number: 613.0994

Published in Australia by
McGraw-Hill Education (Australia) Pty Ltd
Level 2, 82 Waterloo Road, North Ryde NSW 2113
Associate publisher: Sarah Long
Permissions editor: Haidi Bernhardt
Senior production editor: Yani Silvana
Copyeditor: Rosemary Moore
Proofreader: Nicole McKenzie
Indexer: Shelley Barons
Design Coordinator: Dominic Giustarini
Cover design: Astred Hicks, Design Cherry
Interior design: Lauren Statham
Cartoonist: Suzanne Plater
Typeset in Berling 9.5/12 by Laserwords Private Ltd, India
Printed in China on 70 gsm matt art by RR Donnelley

Foreword to the third edition

With its appearance in 1990, the first edition of this book helped to define the field of health promotion strategies and methods. Its balanced approach to individual change, group dynamics, population approaches through mass media and community organisation, and environmental changes through policy initiatives and enforcement earned this book a place in the centre of health promotion. With that balance, it could defend itself in the withering crossfire of the critical, more-rigorous-than-thou scientific reductionism on one side and the rhetoric of the more-equitable-than-thou healthy communities movement on the other.

It could encompass the building-block approach to a health promotion scientifically grounded in theories of health behavioural change and randomised trials that have tested best practices of intervention to change behaviour. At the same time, it offered challenges and experience in broader community interventions and policy changes that could bring about improved conditions of living and environmental supports for people seeking to gain greater control over the determinants of their health. These parameters of the field of health promotion have divided the advocates of opposing ideologically rooted positions and scientifically rigid positions, but their amalgamation in the sweep of this book has made it possible to accommodate both extremes—and the vast middle ground between them.

In the years since the first edition, health promotion has matured scientifically on the behavioural side and has recorded notable successes on the policy and environmental side. The cumulative evidence from patient education and randomised trials of behavioural change has mounted to the point of offering some precision in guidelines for clinical practice of smoking cessation, weight control and other risk factor interventions associated with chronic diseases. At the same time, experience in work sites, schools and communities has been documented with increasing consistency, to provide guidance for public health practitioners and policy makers seeking to bring about changes in media and other environments to make them more conducive to health for whole populations.

This third edition reflects these advances in the now flourishing science and art of health promotion. It encompasses the spectrum of individual, group, institutional, community and societal strategies and methods for which theory, research and experience have provided a growing base of confidence among health promotion planners and practitioners.

LAWRENCE W. GREEN
Professor, Health Care and Epidemiology, Faculty of Medicine
Director, Institute of Health Promotion Research, Faculty of Graduate Studies
University of British Columbia, Vancouver, BC, Canada

Contents

Contents

Acknowledgments

The original edition of this book was based on materials originally developed for the Distance Education Program of the Postgraduate Diploma in Health Promotion at Curtin University of Technology.

The third edition of *Health Promotion Strategies and Methods* would not have been possible without the help of many individuals and organisations. In particular, the authors would like to thank all those who contributed case studies, ideas and suggestions to this edition.

We are grateful for the support and encouragement provided by a number of organisations, including Queensland Health, VicHealth, the Health Department of Western Australia, the Northern Territory Department of Health and Community Services, the Cancer Council of Western Australia and the School of Public Health at Curtin University.

We also wish to acknowledge all the individuals and organisations who contributed to the first and revised editions of this book.

Credits

The publishers would like to express their thanks for permission to reproduce the following items:

Figure 3.1
Copyright 2003 American Diabetes Association
From Diabetes Care®, Vol. 26, 2003; 1186–1192
Reprinted by permission of the American Diabetes Association

Figures 1.1–1.4
Courtesy of the Australian Institute of Health and Welfare

Figure 1.6
The Ottawa Charter for Health Promotion, http://www.who.int/health promotion/conferences/previous/ottawa/en/index4.html, accessed May 2013

p. 228
Courtesy of Dendy Films

About the authors

Professor Garry Egger AM MPH PhD M.A.P.S. has worked in epidemiology and health promotion in government and industry and as a consultant for the World Health Organization and governments in Australasia and South-East Asia since 1971. He started the 'GutBusters' men's waist loss program for men in 1991 and 'Professor Trim's Medically Supervised Weight Loss Programs' in 2003. He has conducted academic training in chronic disease management for Australia's general practitioners. Professor Egger wrote the NH&MRC *Guidelines for Physical Activity* and the *Clinical Guidelines for Weight Control and Obesity Management* for doctors. He has written 30 books (including four textbooks) and several scientific articles. In 1978–80 he ran one of the first major health promotion sentinel studies—the Healthy Lifestyle Project—in New South Wales, after which tobacco advertising was restricted in Australia. Dr Egger has appeared on, or written for, most media outlets, including *60 Minutes, Four Corners, A Current Affair, Today Tonight, The Sydney Morning Herald, The Bulletin* and *The Australian*. He is a council member of the Australian Society for the Study of Obesity (ASSO) and a Fellow of the Australian Council for Health, Physical Education and Recreation (ACHPER). In 2008 he was a foundation member of the Australian Lifestyle Medicine Association (ALMA).

Dr Ross Spark MSc PhD was Director of the Tropical Public Health Unit Network for Queensland Health, based in Cairns, since 1993. He spent most of his career in northern Australia, primarily involved in tropical and Indigenous health issues. As senior research fellow in the School of Public Health at Curtin University, Perth (1989–92), he conducted health promotion research in the Kimberley region. Before that he spent five years as Director of Health Promotion Services with the Northern Territory Department of Health in Darwin. He had undergraduate degrees (BEd, BA) from the University of Queensland, an MSc in public health from the University of Oregon and a PhD from the School of Public Health at Curtin University. He held adjunct academic appointments as associate professor in the School of Public Health at Curtin University, the School of Population

Health at the University of Queensland and the School of Public Health and Tropical Medicine at James Cook University. He also consulted in the Asia–Pacific region in public health and health promotion for AusAID, the Secretariat of Pacific Communities and the World Health Organization. At the time of his death in 2013 he was Professor of Public Health at James Cook University in Cairns.

Rob Donovan PhD (Psychology) is Professor of Behavioural Research in the Faculty of Health Sciences, Adjunct Professor of Social Marketing in the School of Marketing and principal of Mentally Healthy WA's Act-Belong-Commit campaign at Curtin University. A registered psychologist, he has held academic positions in marketing in several US universities and been a Visiting Scientist at the Centers for Disease Control and Prevention in Atlanta, Georgia. He began his marketing career in the marketing department of a major brewery and has had extensive commercial marketing and advertising research experience for a variety of state and national clients. In 1974 he founded Donovan Research, which was absorbed first by NFO WorldWide and is now part of TNS Research. He has an international reputation in social marketing and health promotion, with around 200 (co-authored) books, book chapters and refereed journal articles, and a similar number of technical reports. He has provided expert court testimony on the marketing practices of the tobacco and pharmaceutical industries and served on many state and national committees on a variety of topics. Until recently he was Deputy Chair of the WA Ministerial Council on Suicide Prevention; he is Vice-president of the Board of Relationships Australia WA and a foundation member of the World Anti-Doping Agency's Education Committee. He currently chairs WADA's Social Science Research Ad Hoc Committee.

chapter 1

Towards better health

Summary of main points

* In 2012 Australia had one of the highest life expectancies in the world: 79.5 years for males and 84 years for females. It was also one of the world's wealthiest countries.

* On the negative side, the continuing high levels of certain chronic diseases and poorer health among disadvantaged groups take the edge off improved longevity.

* More than 99 per cent of the population have at least one risk factor for poor health, and 15 per cent have five or more risk factors.

* Obesity rates are among the highest in the Organisation for Economic Co-operation and Development (OECD) countries, and type 2 diabetes associated with this (at around 8% of the population) continues to increase.

* Some infectious diseases that were thought to be a thing of the past have re-emerged and new infectious diseases, some resulting from resistance developed to previously effective treatments, are likely to present challenges in the future (e.g. multiple drug resistant tuberculosis).

* The health of neighbouring Asian and Pacific countries is even more affected by modern industrialised lifestyles as they go through a 'developmental transition'.

* Health promotion is a maturing 'art–science' involving processes of individual, social and environmental change as well as evidence-based health sciences content.

* This book continues to expand on our initial (1990) model of health promotion focusing on strategies and methods aimed at individuals, groups and populations.

Changing health patterns

Overall, the health of people throughout the world, at least as measured by increased longevity and decreased morbidity, has improved dramatically in the last century (Riley 2001; Wang et al. 2012). Still, big differences exist both within and between countries, influenced by changing social, economic and environmental factors and more fixed genetic and cultural factors. In general, and in our region in particular, health patterns in developed countries like Australia and New Zealand need to be considered separately from those of developing nations in Asia and the Pacific, as many of these societies are in a now commonly recognised 'epidemiological transition' (Frenk et al. 1989) from traditional to developed societies.

Such a transition is exemplified by a shift from a predominance of infectious diseases to a rising prominence of chronic diseases, as shown in Figure 1.1. Various analysts have attributed this to 'modernity', 'industrialisation' or causes (broadly called 'anthropogens') associated with 'modern man-made environments, their by-products and/or lifestyles encouraged by those environments' (Egger 2012b). The rise in such diseases has given rise to an interesting phenomenon (see Figure 1.1) where longevity is increased, but more people are living with health-related disabilities (Horton 2012). This suggests that while we might be living *longer*, we may, in many cases, not necessarily be living *better*. Greater emphasis might therefore need to be put on improving health rather than delaying death, thus calling on a greater input from health promotion services.

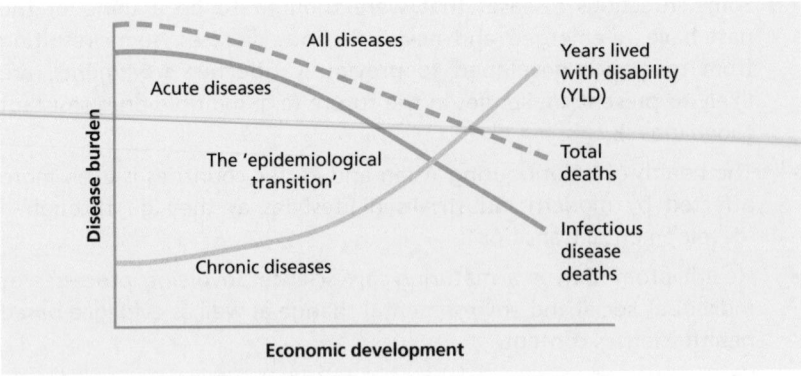

Figure 1.1: Typical changes in patterns of disease with economic development showing the 'epidemiological transition'   AIHW 2012

Health in Australia and New Zealand

Improvements in health in Australia and New Zealand over the twentieth century and first decade of the twenty-first century occurred in several phases. First, there was a period of increases in life expectancy from 1900 to around 1930—largely attributable to improvements in the environment and public health, such as better housing, sanitation and education. The consolidation of the 'germ theory' of disease in the late 1800s helped focus health specialists on a single generic cause of disease: 'germs' or microbial organisms. This led to developments such as immunisation, antibiotics and pasteurisation, as well as to the public health initiatives referred to above, which resulted in the decline in influence on human health of infections through microbial causes.

In a second phase, from the 1930s to the 1970s, there was a levelling of improvements in infectious diseases but the beginnings of a rise in lifestyle-related diseases, which by the mid 1950s had surpassed infectious diseases as the main cause of death (Egger 1978). During a third phase, from 1970 to the end of the first decade of the twenty-first century, there has been a recognition of and greater emphasis on these lifestyle-related diseases, along with an increased appreciation of their socio-environmental aetiologies.

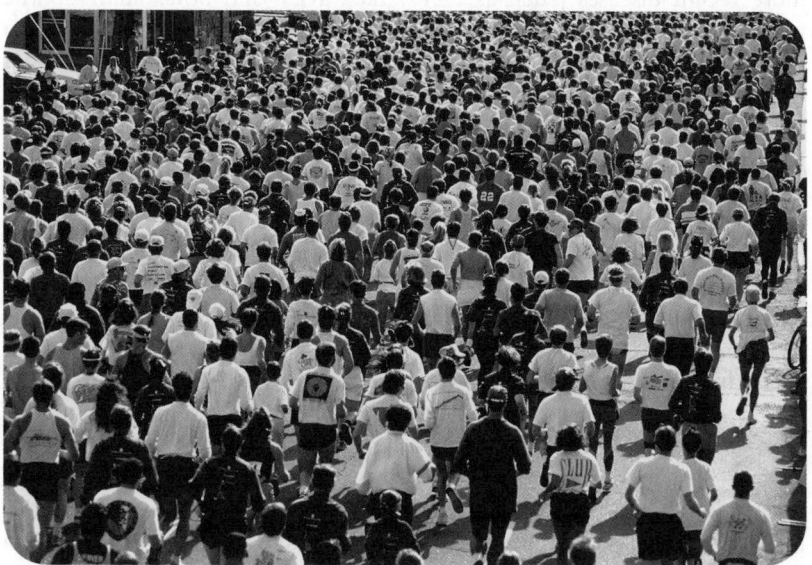

Photo Library

Changing definitions

The change in prominence of different types of disease has led to a confusion of terminology. Initially, a distinction was made between communicable and non-communicable diseases.[1] The 'diseases of modernity' have typically been labelled non-communicable. However, a 2003 World Health Organization (WHO) report suggests that 'chronic conditions' is a better overall term as this encompasses certain communicable diseases (e.g. HIV/AIDS, tuberculosis) which, because of advances in treatment methods, have become chronic health problems, along with other chronic disease such as diabetes, heart disease and cancers, that can't be 'cured' (like acute conditions) but can be 'managed' through organised 'systems of care' to prevent or delay disease complications, sometimes over many years. In chronic disease management, other 'allied' health professionals, as well as the patient, are as vital as the doctor or nurse for effective health outcomes. Chronic conditions also include long-term mental disorders (e.g. depression, schizophrenia) and ongoing structural and physical impairments (e.g. blindness, amputations). 'Chronic' and 'acute' disease are therefore likely to replace earlier terms over time.

A fourth phase now appears to be beginning in which old infectious diseases (such as tuberculosis), newly appearing infectious diseases (or diseases that are spreading to new geographical areas, such as cholera in South America and yellow fever in Kenya), new strains of influenza and more recent diseases (such as HIV/AIDS, avian and other animal-borne influenzas, and medication-resistant disease strains), are emerging as a threat to public health (Heymann & Rodier 2004; ECDPC 2012). Increases in latitude-related diseases associated with climate change are now also becoming more of an accepted reality. Hence there is the potential double jeopardy of rising infections as well as non-infectious diseases in future. As history has shown, infectious diseases still pose an enormous threat to humanity. The great influenza epidemic of 1918, for example, is thought to have killed between 40 million and 100 million people worldwide, and the story of its beginnings and spread is revealing (Barry 2004), with significance for future outbreaks. Currently, prevention, early detection and public health measures remain the best (and only) effective forms of management for such a contingency.

Health promotion needs to be cognisant of and responsive to this changing public health landscape. There is little doubt that the highest priority for health promotion in the early part of the second decade of the twenty-first century is the chronic diseases such as diabetes, heart disease, injury and preventable cancers and their respective risk factors to which, in developed countries like Australia and New Zealand, more than 80 per cent of the burden of disease can be attributed (AIHW 2012). However, many of the strategies and methods of health promotion are, and need to be, equally applicable to an integrated public health response for the management and control of communicable and emerging infectious diseases.

What is 'burden of disease'?

'Burden of disease', or 'BoD', is used to assess and compare the relative impact of different diseases and injuries on people or populations. Burden of disease is used to add the impacts of premature death and prolonged illness or disability for a given disease or injury; it usually uses the disability-adjusted life year (DALY) measure.

AIHW 2012

Despite some concerns for the future, there have been big improvements in life expectancy over time. In fact, Australians now enjoy one of the highest longevities in the world. In *Australia's Health 2012* (AIHW 2012) longevity was reported as being 79.5 years for males and 84 years for females. This puts Australians among the longest living people in the world, exceeded only by the Japanese, Icelanders and Swedish men and French women. Interestingly, the gap between male and female longevity (at one point around 7 years) is also diminishing. In comparison, longevity at the beginning of the twentieth century was around 55 years for Australian men and 59 years for women, indicating a 45 per cent increase over a period of only 100 years. In New Zealand, the figures for the non-Maori population are similar; the improvements for the Maori, as for Indigenous Australians, have not been so impressive. While the health of Indigenous Australians does seem to be improving (male longevity increased to 67 from 55 just a decade ago[2]), it still lags behind health in the non-Indigenous population.

A snapshot of Australia's health, 2012

- The burden of infectious disease has reduced markedly over the past century, from 13 per cent of all deaths in 1907 to 1.3 per cent in 2009.
- Heart disease was still the leading cause of death for both males and females in 2009, followed by lung cancer for males and stroke for females.
- Between 1989–90 and 2007–08, the age-standardised prevalence of diabetes more than doubled, increasing from 1.5 per cent to 4.1 per cent of the Australian population. These are clinically diagnosed cases only. A similar proportion is estimated to be undiagnosed, giving a prevalence rate of around 8 per cent.
- The majority (85%) of Australians aged 15 and over rate their health as 'good' or better, but this assessment decreases with age.
- Over the past 30 years, perinatal mortality rates reduced to almost a quarter of those observed in the 1970s. Rates are now lower in Australia than other comparable developed countries.

continued

continued

- An estimated 222 100 Australians (1%) had dementia in 2011; this is projected to increase to more than 464 000 (1.6%) by 2031.
- Almost 1 in 7 Australians suffer from chronic kidney disease. This has increased more than sevenfold since 1977.
- Forty-five per cent of Australians aged 16–85 have experienced a mental disorder sometime in their lifetime, and about 1 in 9 Australians aged 16–85 have a mental disorder and a physical condition concurrently.
- Although many older Australians have good mental and physical health, nearly half of those aged 65–74 have five or more long-term physical health conditions.
- In 2009, 4 million people in Australia (18.5%) reported having a disability. The prevalence of disability fell from 20 per cent in 2003.
- In 2010, injury was estimated to account for 6.5 per cent of the total burden of disease in Australia, and this is still the leading cause of death for people under 45.
- In 2007–08, 25 per cent of Australian adults (aged 18 and over) and 8 per cent of children (aged 5–17) were obese; this equates to almost 3 million people.

AIHW 2012

Improvements in individual disease categories have also been impressive. For example, there has been a greater than 50 per cent decline in heart disease death rates since 1970, as well as decreases in perinatal mortality, injury, lung cancer, stroke and disability.

No obvious single factor has caused these changes. Improvements in health care are proposed as one factor. But equally, health promotion activities and improvements in prevention techniques, including changes in certain aspects of lifestyle (altered diet, increased exercise, reductions in smoking, changes in motor vehicle driver behaviour), combined with environmental and regulatory interventions, have almost certainly played a part. (For a list of these interventions and their estimated effects, see Appendix A and the box titled 'The returns on investment from health promotion'.)

Still, despite the improvements, there remains considerable opportunity for further improvements in the health of Australians and some concern for the future. For example, the incidence of heart disease in Australia, the UK and the US is still four times that of Japan. Type 2 diabetes is now in epidemic proportions with up to 8 per cent of the population being affected and an estimated additional 16 per cent having what is classified as 'pre-diabetes' and thus likely to develop full-blown diabetes within a decade. Many forms of cancer are still prominent and there is a rise in ailments associated with the increasing ageing of the population such as dementia, Alzheimer disease and injury from falls. Perhaps even more worrying is the

The returns on investment from health promotion

A report in 2003 that projected to 2010 the epidemiological and economic savings made from several major health promotion activities in Australia revealed the following:

- Road safety initiatives—including those encouraging people to wear seatbelts, not drink and drive, and observe speed limits—were saving 1000 lives and about 5000 hospital cases every year.
- Conservatively, between 1970 and 2010, 10 per cent of the decline in tobacco consumption rates can be attributed to health promotion campaigns, with net benefits equalling $2 billion.
- The rate of HIV transmission would have been 25 per cent higher if the national education and prevention campaigns had not been implemented.
- The introduction of subsidised immunisations for measles in 1970 saved an estimated 95 lives and averted about 4 million cases between 1970 and 2003, with net benefits exceeding $9.1 billion.
- The net benefit of campaigns targeting heart disease and associated risk factors between 1970 and 2010 was $1.98 billion.
- Returns to the community were more significant than financial returns to the government.

DHA 2003

rise in ailments associated with a possible deteriorating environment. Both the causes and proposed outcomes of climate change have been implicated in changing aspects of health (McMichael, Montgomery & Costello 2012; Egger & Dixon 2010). There are suggestions that Australia may have reached, or even passed a 'sweet spot' in both health (Egger & Swinburn 2011) and economic prosperity (Harcher 2011), beyond which negative returns might begin to occur in both areas.

A review of evidence has shown major changes in public health since the 1960s and 1970s in Australia. The trends observed since the 1990s are shown in Table 1.1.

Measures of improvement

Another important factor to be considered is the relative emphasis we place on death (mortality) versus illness (morbidity). Historically, medical interventions have focused on treating life-threatening illnesses, which in recent years have been the chronic degenerative diseases—such as stroke, cancer and heart disease. However, we all must die at some time and, in old age, disease leading to rapid death may be viewed as a good to be sought rather than as an evil to be shunned. It is logical, therefore, to place more

Table 1.1: Changes in health and health risks in Australia in recent times (as measured by burden of disease)

Improvements	Mixed changes	Little or no change	Areas getting worse
Overall mortality (particularly infants)	Poor improvements in lower socio-economic groups	Premature births	Diabetes
Heart disease	Chronic respiratory diseases	Asthma	Obesity and related metabolic problems (e.g. diabetes, fatty liver)
Stroke	Heart disease	Physical inactivity	Dementia
Road safety	Lung cancer	Prostate cancer	Arthritis/ musculoskeletal problems
Dental health	Indigenous health	Injury	Depression, mental health
Congenital abnormalities	Cervical cancer	Digestive disorders	Cancer (overall)
Loss of all natural teeth	Skin cancer	Genito-urinary diseases	Health inequalities
Vaccine preventable diseases	Breast cancer		Emerging infectious diseases
Colorectal cancer	Youth suicide		Environmental pollution problems
Breast cancer	Violence		Falls injuries
Smoking	HIV/AIDS		
Cancer survival			

emphasis on preventing the diseases that cause premature death or disability than death per se. One way of doing this is by using a common metric, the disability-adjusted life year, or DALY. One DALY is a lost year of 'healthy life' and is calculated as a combination of years of life lost (YLL) due to premature mortality, and equivalent 'healthy' years lived with disability (YLD). When these are considered, the picture is somewhat different to simple mortality. Figure 1.2 shows the estimated and projected DALYs for major disease categories in 2003 and 2010. From this, and Table 1.1, a different picture of progress emerges: cancer, nervous system and sense

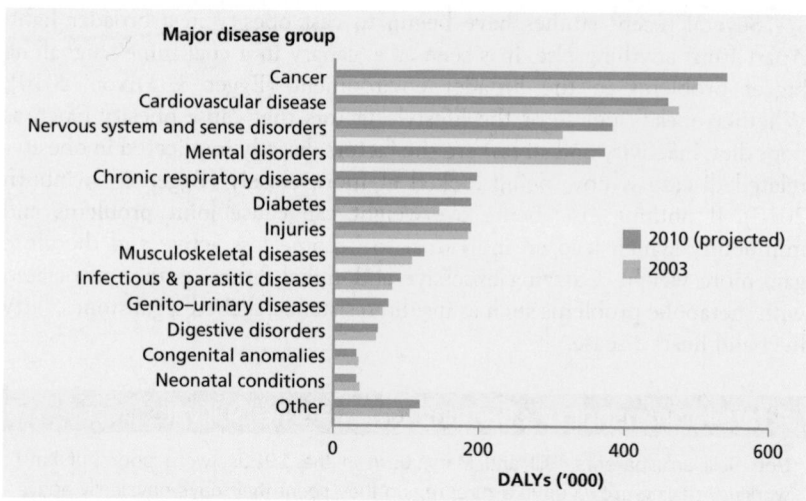

Figure 1.2: Estimated and projected total burden (DALYs) of major disease groups, Australia, 2003 and 2010   AIHW 2012

disorders, mental disorders, diabetes, infectious and parasitic diseases, and musculoskeletal diseases are all increasing in terms of their disease burden, a fact not readily obvious when looking at mortality data.

The rise of obesity

Since the first edition of this text in 1990, obesity has become one of the world's biggest and fastest growing epidemics. Over 67 per cent of Australian men and 55 per cent of women are now overweight or obese, as measured by a body mass index (BMI)[3] of greater than 25: around 25 per cent of Australians are classified as obese, with a BMI >30 (IDI 2009). Weight gain in men over the past decade has averaged around 1.4 g per day and in women around 1.5 g per day (AIHW 2012). In New Zealand the figures are similar, but in the surrounding countries of the Pacific they are even higher (see p.13).

   This would be of little concern if obesity were just an aesthetic issue, but research over the past two decades has shown a growing list of diseases (at least 35) with which obesity is associated. It is now proposed that obesity is the first visible sign of a range of different problems associated with metabolism, variously known as the 'metabolic syndrome', with insulin resistance as an underlying factor. More importantly, the epidemic of obesity appears to have spawned a cascade of smaller epidemics, including diabetes, sleep apnoea, fatty liver, renal failure and joint problems.

Several recent studies have begun to cast obesity in a broader light. Apart from anything else, it is seen as a 'canary in a coal mine', signalling bigger problems in the broader environment (Egger & Dixon 2010). Whether obesity per se or the lifestyle factors that cause obesity (such as poor diet, inactivity and stress) are the factors directly implicated in obesity-related disease is now being looked at more closely (Egger & Swinburn 2010). If nothing else, being overweight can cause joint problems and immobility, which lead an individual to become less active and therefore gain more weight. Carrying excessive abdominal fatness is then associated with metabolic problems such as insulin resistance, diabetes, gallstones, fatty liver and heart disease.

A family snapshot of changing times—'The Sullivans'

Bob Sullivan's parents, Bill and Mary, born in the 1920s, were poor but hard working. Having grown up in a rural region they spent their days physically active in growing and cultivating food for themselves and for sale at the local markets. Such food was 'natural' and healthy, as humans had evolved eating this type of unprocessed product for thousands of years. As a result, Bill and his wife Mary were lean and healthy (although the effects of smoking taken up since World War II were starting to take its effects on Bill and it was a constant battle to avoid serious infections such as polio and diphtheria). They lived into their late 60s, with a short period of illness before death. Bill and Mary's offspring, Bob and Barbara, achieved much greater wealth in their lifetime than Bill and Mary could ever have dreamed possible. As a result they had energy-rich, processed food on the table every day without much (physical) effort. And technology meant they hardly had to lift a finger to enjoy the good life. But around 1980 they started to get fat. As a result, Bob developed type 2 diabetes and Barbara polycystic ovaries. They're still alive in their 70s but Bob has now had a stroke and is confined to a wheelchair. Barbara is also feeling the side effects of the good life and both have had to 'downsize' their living conditions which, they are told, is not good for the economy.

Egger 2012a

One of the ironies of the obesity epidemic is that it exists even in those developing countries where malnutrition is common, because of the presence of high-energy-dense, but low-nutrient-value processed foods. As obesity is a disease of modernisation, related to the increased availability of energy-dense foods and energy-saving technology, it is unlikely to decrease in the short term, at least in the absence of a major crisis such as an economic downturn, oil shortage or war. Infectious disease epidemics of the past, such as smallpox, have taken hundreds of years to overcome. This is despite smallpox and other similar diseases being unpleasant to contract at best, and rapidly fatal at worst. The process of contracting obesity, on the other hand, can be quite pleasant and easy to do (just eat more and move less) and hence is even less likely to be defeated in the short term. In the meantime, the only significant hope is an increase in individual knowledge—given lower rates of the problem among higher educated individuals—and changes in obesity-inducing environments.

Determinants of health

There are many factors that influence health in individuals and populations (see Figures 1.3 and 1.4). Determinants help explain and predict trends in health and explain why some groups have better or worse health than others. They are the key to the prevention of disease, illness or injury. Some determinants, like cigarette smoking, are 'risk factors' whereas others, like healthy food intake, are 'protective factors'. A description of the different types of determinants is shown in the box below.

Levels of health determinants

Drivers are the key linear forces behind disease causality. They range from **proximal** (i.e. more immediate to the disease) to **distal**. Obesity, for example, has proximal drivers of energy over-consumption, medial drivers of obesogenic food environments and distal drivers of economic policies. **Mediators** are influences on the causal pathway (e.g. agricultural subsidies for fat/sugar, lower cost for manufacturing, lower retail prices, increased consumption of high fat/sugar foods). **Moderators** accentuate or attenuate factors on the causal pathway (e.g. the built environment or cultural impacts on health behaviours). **Enablers** are conditions allowing causal factors to be exhibited (e.g. sufficient disposable income to permit over-consumption of food).

Egger, Swinburn & Islam 2012

Behavioural factors can be changed, but biological factors, like age, gender and genes generally cannot (although in the case of the latter, much work is currently being carried out to use genetic knowledge to treat and counsel prospective parents regarding diseases with a genetic basis). Since its mapping in 2001, the human genome is now focusing medical research on genetic 'cures' for a range of different problems, with exciting prospects for the future, although to date the outcomes have been modest. Genetic screening is well under way and the future is likely to see more individualised approaches such as dietary prescription through psycho–pharmaco–genomic techniques. Gene mapping of the human biome (biological organisms making up those that live on and within the human body) is also likely to yield new interventions in the future.

As shown in Figure 1.3, a relatively small number of risk factors accounts for a significant proportion of diseases.

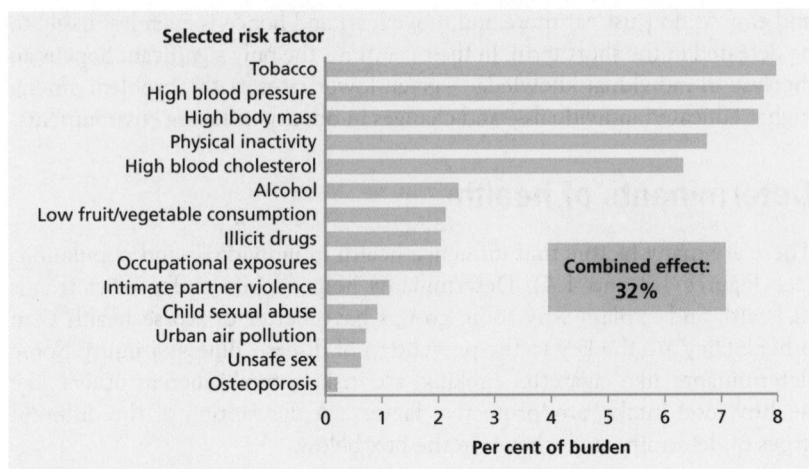

Figure 1.3: **Burden of disease from 14 selected risk factors**   AIHW 2012

Determinants have been described as a web of causes with broad causal pathways or 'chains' that affect health (AIHW 2012), as is shown in Figure 1.4.

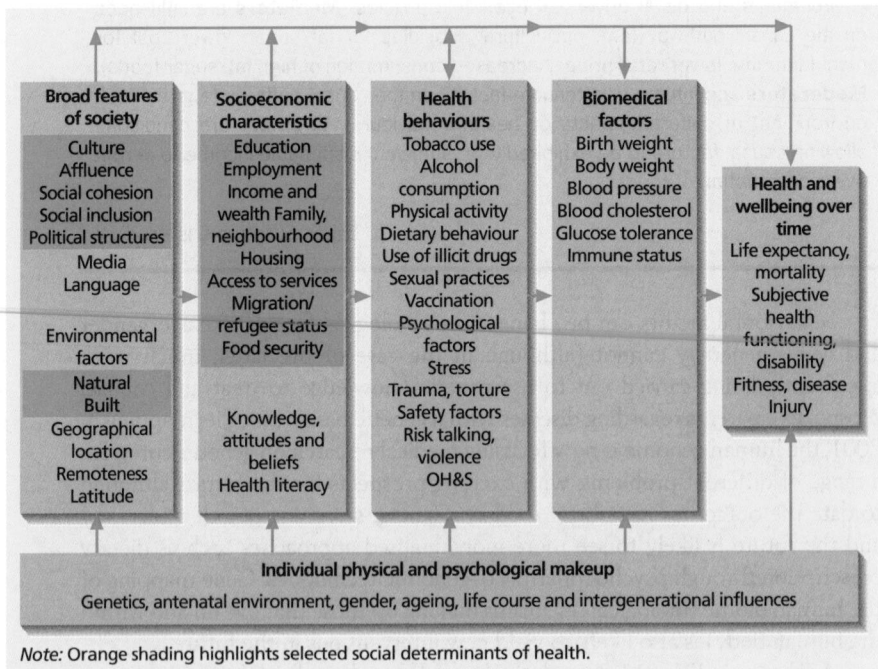

Note: Orange shading highlights selected social determinants of health.

Figure 1.4: **A framework for the determinants of health**   AIHW 2012

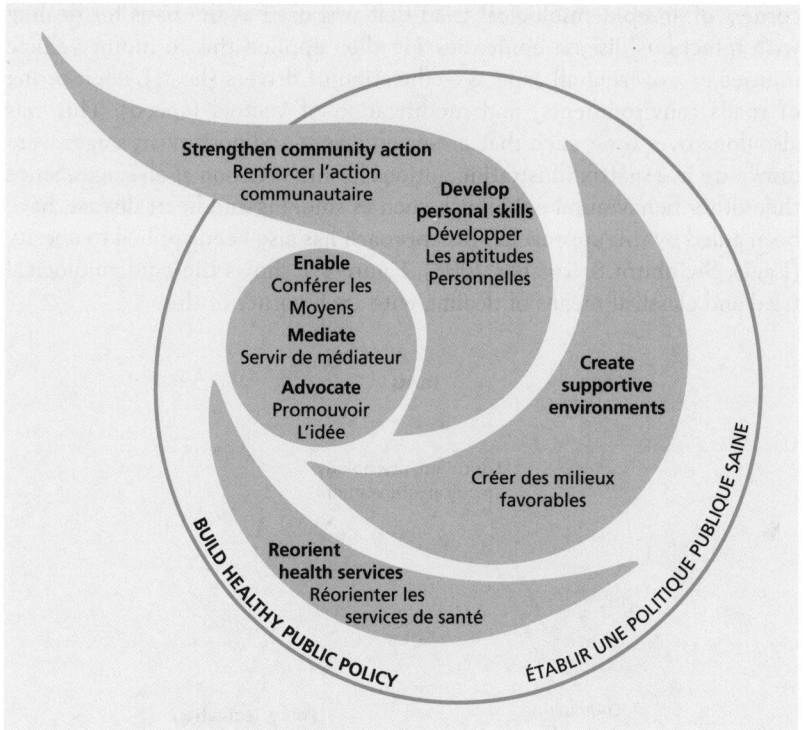

Figure 1.6: The health promotion emblem   WHO 2009

its nature, is orientated to the individual. However, early writings from the 1970s and beyond changed the emphasis to a wider scale requiring socio-political attributions and the involvement of a number of different disciplines. For example, the Lalonde report in 1974 (Green et al. 1980) introduced into public policy the notion that all causes of death and disease have four contributing elements:

- inadequacies of the existing healthcare system
- behavioural factors and unhealthy lifestyles
- environmental hazards
- human biological factors.

The central message of the Lalonde report was that improvements in environments and in the lifestyles of individuals would be the single most effective means of reducing mortality and morbidity.

The 1970s also saw a paradigm shift in thinking in relation to prevention when an American engineer, Dr William Haddon, applied a traditional epidemiological approach to what was considered an intractable problem—injury (Haddon 1980). Haddon recognised the importance of the host, vector and environment, which had for years made up the three corners of an epidemiological triad that was used as the basis for dealing with infectious disease epidemics. He then applied this to motor vehicle injuries by covering all aspects—education of drivers (hosts), engineering of roads (environments) and modification of vectors (speed). This was also done over time, such that pre-event, event and post-event stages were drawn up in a matrix illustrating options for intervention at all stages. Since then other behavioural epidemics, such as smoking and heart disease, have been aided by this approach. This approach has also been applied to obesity (Egger, Swinburn & Rossner 2003). Figure 1.7 shows the epidemiological triad and classical means of dealing with each corner of this.

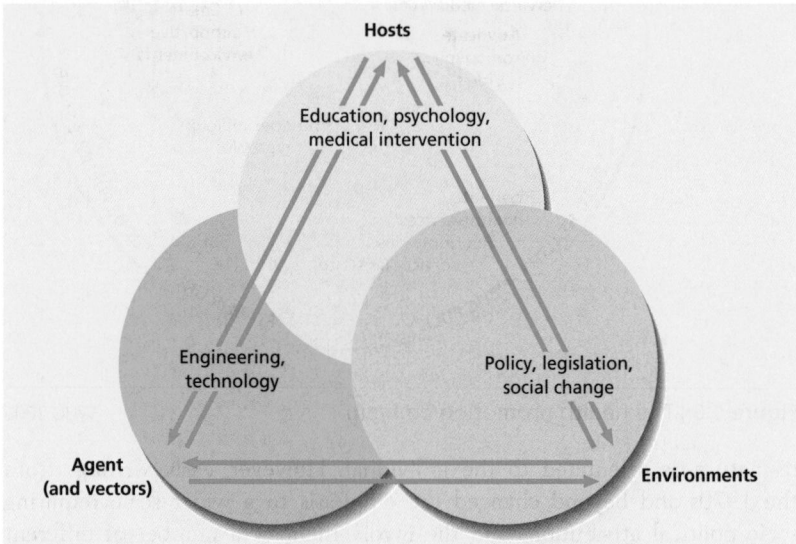

Figure 1.7: The epidemiological triad and approaches to dealing with each corner

These early initiatives were followed by the Ottawa Charter for Health Promotion in 1986, which outlined five specific actions for health promotion under a new public health. These were:

- developing healthy public policy
- developing personal skills
- strengthening community action
- creating supportive environments
- re-orienting health services.

A further five international charters, regulations or conferences on health promotion occurred up to 2005. These all identified and slightly modified actions, commitments and pledges associated with health promotion, culminating in the report *Milestones in Health Promotion* published in 2009 (WHO 2009).

A framework for health promotion

As a relatively new field, health promotion has yet to achieve a universally agreed upon framework of operation for achieving the goals specified above. Indeed, this may not be possible given the dynamic nature of the profession. There is, however, a range of approaches currently used (including the epidemiological triad described previously), varying in focus from dealing with specific health issues (e.g. smoking, drug use, inactivity, weight loss) to focusing on 'settings' (e.g. schools, workplaces, villages) and 'sectors' (e.g. industries, government agencies), or even broader social change (e.g. political and economic action to reduce health inequalities).

Figure 1.8 presents a framework on which the structure of this text is based. We have chosen to focus on individuals, groups or populations to demonstrate the strategies and tools of health promotion practitioners. The strategies range from educational and motivational approaches, and social marketing techniques, to economic, regulatory, technological and organisational interventions. The first two of these primarily address intra- and inter-personal factors underlying risks for health, whereas the last four are aimed at the socio-political, physical or socio-cultural environments—addressing the 'risk conditions' for health. Although these strategies can be used singly, research indicates that health promotion interventions are more likely to be effective where combinations of strategies are employed (WHO 2009).

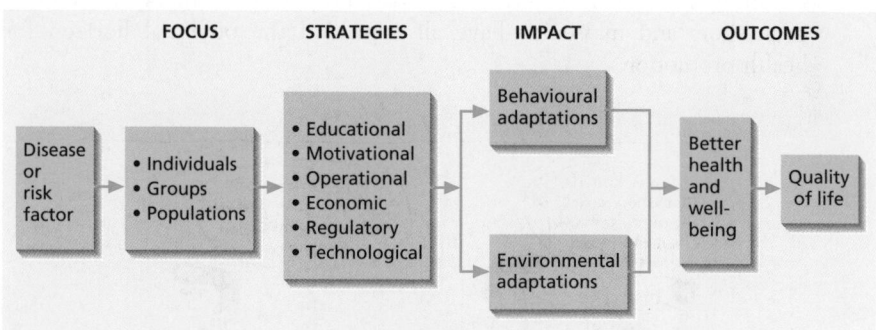

Figure 1.8: A framework for health promotion

The role of the health promotion practitioner

Health promotion, as an emerging discipline, has been clouded by competing philosophies and theories, by battles for professional territory, and by fights for government funds. Different players in this game have been adversely labelled as following a *medical* model or, equally adversely, as following an unscientific *social or political* model. This has sometimes led to a dilemma of professional identity for those working in the field.

In the past, health promotion practitioners have been drawn from a variety of different backgrounds: social and behavioural sciences, medicine, politics, nursing, social welfare and community development. Indeed, many of these disciplines regard health promotion as a small but significant part of their ambit. The advent of specialist tertiary training in health promotion is beginning to define more clearly the role of the full-time health promotion practitioner. Yet the diversity of professional backgrounds from which people come to health promotion remains one of the strengths of this field. We take the view that health promotion is both an art and a science. For example, determining health risk requires a rigorous scientific approach, whereas communicating that risk information is both an art and a science.

The modern health promotion practitioner is now most likely to be part of an interdisciplinary team with a common goal of increasing total health and wellbeing, and decreasing illness in individuals and the broader community. It is not enough that health promotion practitioners be knowledgeable about matters that influence the individual's health; their responsibilities also are to modify the health environment. The advent of organised networks of primary healthcare providers and better government provisions for team care arrangements in chronic disease management have increased the scope for health promotion both within different disciplines and as a discipline itself. New professions—such as life coaches, practice nurses, nurse practitioners and health coaches, and professional sub-disciplines such as physicians' assistants, exercise therapists, dietary counsellors and masseurs—have all expanded the potential horizon for health promotion.

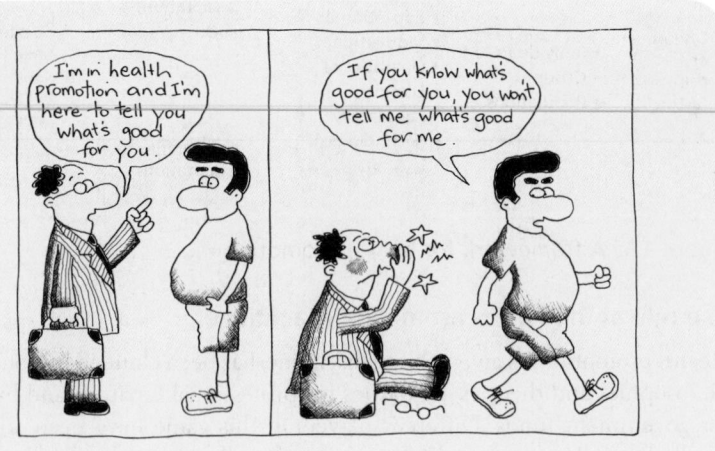

To achieve the requirements of modern health promotion the professional health promotion practitioner needs to be skilled in both *process* and *content*. Historically, the emphasis has been on the body of health information to be communicated—that is, on *content*. Equally important are the means of influencing desired change—that is, *process*. For example, to improve a community's health through changes in nutrition requires an ability to use processes to influence dietary behaviour in line with the content of scientific information available on the benefits of such a change and in the context of broader socio-cultural influences.

Unlike the science of medicine, where a drug discovery can have a continuing impact on health for many years and where clinical areas are becoming more and more specialised, health promotion needs to monitor and respond to the dynamically changing needs, attitudes, fears and mores of a society. Because health promotion programs take time to plan and put into action, the health promotion practitioner must not only be aware of the community's current trends, but also must possess an ability to chart the direction in which these are likely to move in the future. To this extent health promotion is both art and science. Determining health risk is a science. Communicating that risk information is an art.

Strategies and methods in health promotion

A *strategy* in health promotion as described in the rest of this text is 'a plan of action that anticipates barriers and resources in relation to achieving a specific objective' (Green & Kreuter 1991). A *method* is a tactic employed as part of a strategy. Methods describe the means by which change is to be brought about within the target group. Although some writers use the terms *methods* and *strategies* interchangeably, there are distinctions that are relevant to the understanding of the development of health promotion programs.

Strategies

Strategies can be broad-based—such as introducing regulatory changes conducive to healthy behaviour—or relatively narrowly focused—such as changing workplace smoking policy. Within these strategies, there may be a number of methods of achieving the goals of improved health.

Currently, there are two major strategy dichotomies that have influenced the practice of health promotion. The *first* concerns the emphasis on socio-environmental change versus individual change. The *second* concerns the emphasis on high-risk individuals versus whole populations—where risk is averaged out.

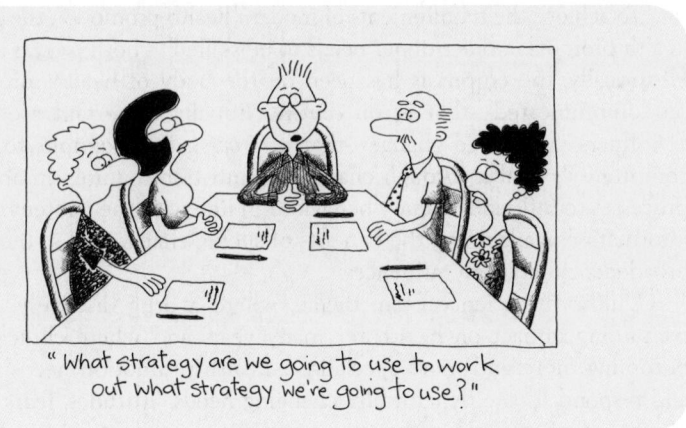

" What strategy are we going to use to work
out what strategy we're going to use?"

Socio-environmental versus individual behavioural strategies

The socio-environmental versus individual behaviourist debate concerns notions of the role of the individual in determining his/her health in contrast to the effect of broader environmental influences.

The *socio-environmental interpretation* places the blame for illness among disadvantaged groups on their comparative social and economic deprivation. Strategies for dealing with this are seen as addressing the causes of this deprivation—causes such as poverty, lack of education, unemployment and social factors. This involves 'targeting the system' rather than 'blaming the victim'.

The *individual interpretation* places emphasis on the responsibility of the individual for his/her health status. According to this view, health-compromising behaviour by individuals is the main factor causing ill-health. This is based on epidemiological studies, which show that most premature death from the major non-communicable diseases (such as heart disease, cancer and stroke) may be attributed to lifestyle factors—known as risk factors. These include smoking, high-fat diets, hypertension, inactivity and stress. This approach suggests that individuals adopt health-compromising behaviours because they have inadequate information, a lack of skills or a negative attitude. The strategies called for here are programs aimed at changing individual behaviour—without specific emphasis on structural factors that may be seen as underlying the causes of behaviour.

In reality, both approaches should be incorporated into programs based on a population perspective (Sallis & Owen 1996; Egger & Swinburn 1996). This synthesis approach focuses attention on both individual and socio-environmental factors as targets for health promotion interventions. It addresses the importance of interventions directed at changing interpersonal, organisational, community and public policy factors that support and maintain healthy behaviours. The approach assumes that appropriate changes in the social environment will produce changes in individuals, and that the support of individuals in the population is essential for implementing environmental changes.

High risk versus low risk (or population-level) strategies

The high risk versus low risk debate was sparked by the famous English epidemiologist Dr Geoffrey Rose (1992), who asked the question: 'Should we be dealing with sick individuals or sick populations?' In essence, the question implies that 'a large number of people at a small risk may give rise to more cases of disease than a small number who are at high risk'. This is also known as 'the prevention paradox'. The corresponding strategies are:

- the *high risk* approach—which seeks to protect susceptible individuals
- the *population*-level approach—which seeks to control the causes of incidence in populations and seeks to shift the whole distribution of exposure in a population. These populations can be regional or national, or specific sub-populations such as older people, women or Aboriginal and Torres Strait islander peoples (AIHI 2012).

According to Rose (1992), 'the two approaches are not usually in competition, but the prior concern should always be to discover and control the causes of incidence'.

A combined high and low risk approach is, in most circumstances and with respect to most health issues, the preferred option. The main principles and strategies for health promotion in this respect include the following components:

- altering the characteristics of lifestyle and environment that are the underlying causes of mass disease (prevention in populations)
- preventing the development in low-incidence countries of these precursors (primary prevention in populations)
- within a population, identifying and helping individuals at special risk (high risk strategy), as well as preventing progression of disease (secondary prevention).

More than two decades after Geoffrey Rose challenged epidemiological thinking, his ideas are still relevant to contemporary public health practice. In a review, Doyle, Furey & Flowers (2006) asserted that individual and population-level approaches are fundamentally different but both are needed. Recent examples of powerful population-level approaches such as tobacco control and the regulation of the food industry prove Rose's point that norms can change, benefitting the most deprived. Individual approaches have also succeeded, despite the fact that ensuring regular uptake by individuals of screening and primary prevention is demanding, and their protection of the most deprived individuals is limited. These authors caution however that the rise of more assertive consumerism in health (e.g. fluoridation and immunisation programs being opposed by groups who are not persuaded of the benefit to others for the risk they (wrongly) perceive to themselves) may put at risk public health initiatives that rely on individual choice alone.

The strategies covered in this book will consider individuals, groups and populations. Within these three areas there is a wide range of methods available for the implementation of health promotion programs. It should be stressed that effective health promotion *requires* this variety of methods; for example, the more complex the concept, the wider the range of methods that may be needed to apply the concept. In essence, the health promotion practitioner needs to be a 'specialist in generalisation' with some knowledge of the content (and knowledge of where to seek out greater content expertise and information), as well as knowledge of a wide variety of the processes involved in delivering such content.

Methods

Methods are tactics by which change is brought about within a target group. For example, community development and mass media are two methods used to describe a host of activities aimed at modifying health behaviour within the realm of community strategies.

Activities are the specific applications of the methods selected. For example, whereas electronic media may be a *method* used to effect a change in community behaviour, the production of a poster, a video or a television commercial would be *activities* using this method.

Some health promotion practitioners may choose to specialise in certain methods—indeed, there is a case for encouraging this to capitalise on and develop specialist talents. However, there should be an acknowledgement that this does not imply that any one method is inherently superior, or can be applied equally, to all health promotion situations.

Career opportunities in health promotion

There has been an expansion of opportunities in health promotion in recent years as a result of the greater emphasis on preventable causes of disease. This has meant not only the advent of health promotion as a profession, but the inclusion of health promotion skills to the roles of other health professionals such as doctors, nurses, occupational therapists, dentists, teachers, dietitians, exercise specialists, psychologists, and many more, now including the sub-specialties such as exercise therapists, dietary aides and masseurs. Changes in roles means that employment possibilities can range from clinical practice in the various professions to work in state and federal health and sport and recreation departments or local government, to work in segments of the private sector such as health insurance, hospitals, advertising, food or fitness. At the international level, the World Health Organization, Secretariat of the Pacific Community, AUSAID, welfare and other aid groups, and private sector organisations, all require personnel with health promotion expertise.

Notes

1. The terms 'communicable' and 'infectious' have often been used interchangeably, although strictly speaking this is not correct. For example, some infectious diseases (such as tetanus) may not be communicable (i.e. transmissible from person to person), whereas communicable diseases are, by definition, always infectious and transmissible.
2. These findings may be spurious, however, because of the increase in numbers of Australians who now identify as being Indigenous.
3. Body mass index is measured by weight (in kilograms) divided by height (in metres^2).

Appendix A: Selected history of health promotion activities in Australia

Educational and behavioural campaigns

1978: 'Quit. For Life' campaign trialled as part of the North Coast Healthy Lifestyle Campaign. Consolidated. Quit campaigns were launched as part of the National Tobacco Strategy 1997–2005.

1978: 'Life. Be In It' campaign receives national funding from the Australian Government.

1980: 'How Will You Go When You Sit for the Test?' campaign to introduce random breath testing in New South Wales.

1981: 'Slip! Slop! Slap!' campaign introduced by Cancer Council Australia. The message was modified to 'Slip! Slop! Slap! Seek! Slide!' in 2007.

1987: 'Grim Reaper' campaign launched—a graphic television campaign aimed at shocking the Australian public into discussions around HIV transmission.

1989: Heart Foundation launches the 'Tick' campaign: a way of helping consumers make heart-healthy food choices.

1997: National Tobacco Campaign: 'Every Cigarette Is Doing You Damage' launched. The campaign is recognised as a leading health promotion campaign worldwide, with material used in more than 42 countries.

2005: 'Go for 2&5TM' released—a national campaign encouraging Australians to increase their daily consumption of fruit and vegetables.

2008: 'Don't Turn a Night Out into a Nightmare' introduced as part of the National Binge Drinking Campaign. The campaign specifically targets children and young adults aged 13–25, as well as parents of children aged 13–17.

2010 and beyond: The Healthy and Active Australia initiative begins, which includes the 'Get Set 4 Life—Healthy Habits for Healthy Kids', 'Healthy Spaces and Places', 'Measure Up' and 'Swap it, Don't Stop It' campaigns.

Current anti-smoking campaigns include 'Who Will You Leave Behind?', 'Break the Chain' targeting Indigenous smokers, and 'Every Cigarette You Don't Smoke Is Doing You Good', which is produced in a variety of languages to target people from culturally and linguistically diverse backgrounds.

Policy and regulation

1953: After the passing of the State Grants (Milk for School Children) Act, all states and territories provide free milk to children aged 13 or under in school.

1953: Fluoridated water is first introduced to Australia in Beaconsfield, Tasmania.

1956: The poliomyelitis (polio) vaccine is introduced to Australia. Mass vaccinations are conducted in primary schools across the country.

1968: Seat belt legislation introduced.

1973: All states and territories require wearing of fitted seatbelts in motor vehicles and helmets for motorcycle riders and passengers.

1981: Drink-driver restrictions brought in with random breath testing.

1986: The first International Conference on Health Promotion was held in Ottawa, Canada. At this conference the Ottawa Charter was developed to achieve Health for All by the year 2000 and beyond.

1990: Bicycle helmet legislation introduced in all states.

1992: All home swimming pools required to have protective fencing to prevent child drowning.

1992: First dietary guidelines published.

1998: Immunise Australia Program launched by the Australian Government, including television advertisements, financial incentives and regulations for school attendance.

2006: National Close the Gap campaign launched to reduce Indigenous health inequality by closing the health and life expectancy gap between Aboriginal and Torres Strait Islander peoples and non-Indigenous Australians within a generation.

2009: Mandatory standards developed requiring the addition of folic acid to bread-making flour, and iodine to bread via iodised salt.

2011: Laws are passed mandating that all tobacco products sold in Australia need to be in plain packaging from 1 December 2012.

Adapted from AIHW: *Australia's Health 2012*

References

AIHI (Australian Indigenous Health Infonet), Working paper, May 2012, p. 10.

AIHW (Australian Institute of Health and Welfare), 2012, *Australia's Health 2012*, Australia's health series no. 13, Cat. no. AUS 156, AIHW, Canberra.

Alcorn, T., & Ouyan, Y., 2012, Diabetes saps health and wealth from China's rise, *Lancet* 379:2227–8.

Barry J.M., 2004, *The Great Influenza: The Epic Story of the Greatest Plague in History*, Penguin, NY.

Brown, J.B, Nichols, G.A, Glauber, H.S, Bakst, A.W., Schaeffer, M., & Kelleher, C.C., 2001, Health care costs associated with escalation of drug treatment in type 2 diabetes mellitus, *Am J Health Syst Pharm* 58(2):151–7.

DHA (Department of Health and Ageing), 2003, *Returns on Investment in Public Health: An Epidemiological and Economic Analysis*, DHA, Canberra.

Doyle, Y.G., Furey, A., & Flowers, J., 2006, Sick individuals and sick populations: 20 years later, *J Epidemiol Community Health* 60:396–8.

Du, S., Lu, B., Zhai, F., & Popkin, B.M., 2002, A new stage of the nutrition transition in China, *Public Health Nutr* 5(1A):169–74.

Egger, G., 1978, Medical nemesis and economic health or economic nemesis and medical health: the modern dilemma, *Aust J Soc Issues* 13(4):287–301.

Egger, G., 2012a, Health and sustainability, in Murray, J., Dey, C., & Andrew, C. (Eds), *The Educator's Guide to Sustainability*, Common Ground, Sydney.

Egger, G., 2012b, In search of a germ theory equivalent for chronic disease, *Prev Chronic Dis* 9(11):1–7.

Egger, G.J., & Dixon, J.B., 2010, Obesity and global warming: are they similar 'canaries' in the same 'mineshaft'?, *Med J Aust* 193(11–12):635–7.

Egger, G., & Swinburn B., 1996, An ecological model for understanding the obesity pandemic, *BMJ* 20: 227–31.

Egger, G., & Swinburn, B., 2010, *Planet Obesity: How We Are Eating Ourselves and the Planet to Death*, Allen & Unwin, Sydney.

Egger, G., & Swinburn, B., 2011, Finding the sweet spot between climate change, human health, and economic growth, *Solutions* 2(5):31–5.

Egger, G., Swinburn, B., & Islam, A., 2012, Economic growth and obesity: a dynamic relationship with interesting implications, *Econ Human Biol* 10(2):147–53.

Egger, G., Swinburn, B., & Rossner, S., 2003, Dusting off the epidemiological triad: could it apply to obesity, *Obes Rev* 4(2):115–20.

Engelgau, M.M., Geiss, L.S., Saaddine, J.B., Boyle, J.P., Benjamin, S.M., Gregg, E.W., Tierney, E.F., Rios-Burrows, N., Mokdad, A.H., Ford, E.S., Imperatore, G., & Venkat Narayan, KM., 2004, The evolving diabetes burden in the United States, *Ann Intern Med* 140(11):945–50.

ECDPC (European Centre for Disease Prevention and Control), 2012, *Communicable Disease Threats Report*, ECDPC, Stockholm.

Frenk, J., Bobadilla, J.L., Sepulveda, J., & Lopez Cervantes, M., 1989, Health transition in middle-income countries: new challenges for health care, *Health Policy and Planning* 4(1):29–39.

Green, L.W. & Kreuter, M.W., 1991, *Health Promotion Planning: An Educational and Environmental Approach*, Mayfield Publishing Co., Mountain View.

Green, L.W., Kreuter, M.W., Deeds, S.G. & Partridge, K.B., 1980, *Health Education Planning: A Diagnostic Approach*, Mayfield Publishing Co., Palo Alto.

Haddon, W., 1980, Advances in the epidemiology of injuries as a basis for public policy, *Public Health Rep* 95:411–21.

Harcher, P., 2011, *The Sweet Spot: How Australia Made Its Own Luck – And Could Now Throw It All Away*, Black Inc, Melbourne.

Heymann, D.L., & Rodier, G., 2004, Global surveillance, national surveillance, and SARS, *Emerg Infect Dis* 10(2): 173–5.

Horton, R., 2012, GBD 2010: understanding disease, injury, and risk, *Lancet* (380):2053–4.

Hu, F.B., Manson, J.E., Stampfer, M.J., Colditz, G., Liu, S., Solomon, C.G., & Willett, W.C., 2001, Diet, lifestyle, and the risk of type 2 diabetes mellitus in women, *N Engl J Med* 345(11):790–7.

IDI (International Diabetes Institute), 2009, *Diabetes in Australia*, IDI and National Health and Medical Research Council, Melbourne.

Marmot, M., & Wilkinson R. 2005, *Social Determinants of Health*, Oxford University Press, London.

McMichael, T., Montgomery, H., & Costello, A., 2012, Health risks, present and future, from global climate change, *BMJ* Mar 19;344:e1359.

Riley, J.C., 2001, *Rising Life Expectancy: A Global History*, Cambridge University Press, New York.

Rose, G., 1992, *The Strategy of Preventive Medicine*, Oxford University Press, Oxford.

Sallis, J.& Owen, N., 1996, Ecological models, In Glantz, K., Lewis, F.M. & Rimer, B.K. (Eds), *Health Behaviour and Health Education: Theory and Practice* (2nd edn), Jossey-Bass, San Francisco, pp. 403–24.

Secretariat of Pacific Communities, 2002, *Obesity in the Pacific: Too Big to Ignore*, SPC Publication, Noumea.

Wang, H., Dwyer-Lindgren, L., Lofgren, K.T., et al., 2012, Age-specific and sex-specific mortality in 187 countries, 1970–2010: a systematic analysis for the Global Burden of Disease Study 2010, *Lancet* (380):2071–94.

WHO (World Health Organization), 2003, *Diet, Food Supply and Obesity in the Pacific*, WA 695, WHO, Geneva.

WHO (World Health Organization), 2009, *Milestones in Health Promotion*, WHO, Geneva.

Wilkinson, R., & Pickett, K., 2010, *The Spirit Level: Why Greater Equality Makes Societies Stronger*, Bloomsbury Press, New York.

Zimmet, P., Shaw, J., & Alberti, K.G., 2003, Preventing type 2 diabetes and the dysmetabolic syndrome in the real world: a realistic view, *Diabet Med* 20(9):693–702.

chapter 2

Health and human behaviour

Summary of main points

- Knowledge of the negative consequences of risky behaviours is generally not sufficient to motivate cessation of unhealthy behaviours and adoption of healthy alternatives.

- Various models of attitude and behaviour change have been proposed to explain and describe people's decision making.

- These models are generally based on people's beliefs about the consequences of behaving in certain ways, their evaluation of these consequences, beliefs about others' endorsement or otherwise of such behaviours, beliefs about the costs and benefits of alternative behaviours, and beliefs about their capabilities in adopting the healthy alternatives.

- The models provide frameworks for formative research, communication strategies and broader interventions.

- The strategies following from these models can be applied to individuals in one-on-one situations, to groups of varying sizes, to intermediaries such as policy makers, and to larger populations through mass media and other channels.

The practical value of theory

It's been said that there's nothing more practical than a good theory. Since one goal of health promotion is to change behaviour, an understanding of the behaviour change process is essential if health promotion strategies are to succeed. Human behaviour, and especially health behaviour, is complex and not always readily understandable. Many theories have been devised in an attempt to explain behaviour. Some are relevant to the study of health, some are not (see Nutbeam & Harris 2004). There is still no unifying theory that comfortably encompasses all those aspects of human behaviour that go to explain health. Indeed, some theories are contradictory and lead to different conclusions under different circumstances. Methods of facilitating behaviour change have also had mixed results.

Because part of the role of the health promotion practitioner is to motivate people towards patterns that will enhance their health, it is important that these theoretical frameworks, however imperfect, are understood and utilised in the selection of strategies and methods. In particular, the practitioner should have a working knowledge of factors that motivate behaviour.

What motivates health behaviour?

Intentions to adopt healthy behaviour, like any other type of behaviour, are motivated or 'triggered' by stimuli in an individual's environment. However, individual responses to such stimuli might or might not relate to health enhancement. For example, the inability to climb a set of stairs without puffing might encourage one individual to seek a higher level of fitness, but encourage another to look for the lifts.

Similarly, health-enhancing behaviours might be adopted for motivations other than to improve health. For example, it is generally believed that more than 60 per cent of those who start an exercise program do so for aesthetic reasons—to lose weight, look good or shape up. Interestingly, those who continue to exercise (only about a third of those who start will continue for longer than three months) tend do so for social and wellbeing reasons rather than physical health reasons (Donovan & Francas 1990).

This opens a second dimension to motivation for health behaviour: the fact that it is dynamic, not static, and might reflect the stage an individual has achieved in adopting and developing a type of behaviour, and that extensive research with target audiences is essential to identify appropriate motivators.

Health knowledge and behaviour

It was a common belief among health professionals—and still is among some—that knowledge about what influences health would be sufficient to motivate individuals towards healthy behaviour. However, the fact that knowledge is neither a necessary nor a sufficient condition for behaviour change is obvious from the fact that the deleterious aspects of smoking are almost universally known but about 20 per cent of the Australian population continues to smoke. Knowledge does not always motivate logically appropriate behaviour. Why?

First, individuals are bombarded with an enormous amount of information or 'clutter' in modern society. Each individual perceives this according to their own psychological predisposition. Individuals can select or ignore those things they don't wish to see or hear—because of anxiety or defences that have been built up to that message—and selectively focus on information that supports their existing beliefs and behaviour. For example, a heavy smoker might go to the refrigerator during an anti-smoking television advertisement rather than face the anxiety that it might cause, and seize on any media reports that question the validity of the link between smoking and lung cancer.

Second, incoming information is interpreted in terms of personal experiences, background, beliefs, values and attitudes. For example, information about the link between smoking and lung cancer can be discounted by smokers who remind themselves of older smokers they know who 'lived to a ripe old age', by arguing that the link is 'only statistical', or by deluding themselves that 'if it was really that bad the government would ban it'; in other words, by rationalising their actions.

Third, the input received and analysed must have personal relevance to the individual for action to be taken; that is, information that a particular diet has benefit for weight control is of little value to someone who does not want to lose weight, or who does not know someone who wants to lose weight.

Finally, even where individuals accept that their behaviour puts them at risk and have a full understanding of subsequent harms, other individual beliefs or environmental factors might inhibit adoption of healthy alternatives. A smoker might be experiencing a stressful period in her life and believe smoking is necessary to help her cope. A single father might believe that fast foods and sweets are nutritionally deficient and 'bad' for his children, but might prefer to give in to the child's demands rather than create conflict in the household. A woman might be convinced that 30 minutes of walking on most days would be beneficial to her health, but put off because the neighbourhood is busy with traffic during the day, the area is poorly lit at night and the footpaths are in poor condition.

In summary, then:

- In some cases, knowledge might be sufficient to elicit changes in behaviour, but in other cases, it might be neither necessary nor sufficient.
- Where knowledge is deemed important, this should be couched in terms relevant to the target audience.
- The transfer of knowledge into action is dependent on a wide range of internal and external factors, including attitudes and beliefs and the physical environment.
- For most individuals, the translation of knowledge into behaviour requires the development of specific skills (enabling factors), which could include interpersonal skills (e.g. parenting communication ability).

Attitudes, values and behaviour

To be acted on, knowledge needs to be incorporated by individuals in a way that both influences—and is influenced by—their personal attitudes and values with respect to health and health-enhancing behaviours. An individual's values affect a wide range of thought and behaviour patterns, in part by generating attitudes. Values precede attitudes in a manner that moves from the general to the specific; that is, a slim figure is prized by many in today's society and this can predispose someone to act positively towards a weight-control program. Similarly, social justice and equity values can lead to positive attitudes towards specific programs targeting disadvantaged children or people with disabilities. Bringing values and attitudes into the equation helps to explain the knowledge–action gap in many instances. Clearly, most people are at ease when the knowledge they hold is consistent with their attitudes and values. If discord arises (known as cognitive dissonance; discussed below), the facts are often interpreted (or misinterpreted) such that the contradiction between knowledge and attitudes is removed. Just as there is no clear association between knowledge and behaviour, there is no guaranteed clear progression from attitudes to behaviour.

In most cases, attitude change precedes forming an intention to change, and thence behavioural change. In many cases, however, behaviour change could precede, and influence, attitudes. For example, many people initially opposed to wearing seat belts became more favourable after the behaviour became compulsory; attitudes to drinking alcohol and driving changed after the introduction of random breath testing.

Maslow's hierarchy of needs

According to Maslow (1968), behaviour is motivated by a hierarchy of human needs (Figure 2.1). At the base of this hierarchy is the desire to satisfy physiological needs: life's sustainers, such as food, water, oxygen and sleep. Once these are met, safety needs are next in the hierarchy, including the need for protection from harm and the alleviation of physical threat. Belongingness and love come next and, once these are satisfied, the need for self-esteem emerges as a primary motivator. Maslow's major contribution to health behaviour theory is his postulated highest level of need—the desire for 'self-actualisation'—which reflects a desire to achieve the full capacity of one's abilities and the self-satisfaction that accompanies it. In practice, Maslow's theory clarifies for the health promotion practitioner why not everybody responds to the practitioner's 'obviously beneficial' and well-meaning interventions. For the low-income single parent, burdened with childcare responsibilities and with little prospect of doing more than just coping from day to day, the lure of a decrease in some forms of behaviour—which aid in the desire for belonging or identity (i.e. drinking alcohol or smoking tobacco)—for the promise of an intangible increase in health is hardly enticing. Health needs in this case might be compromised for the sake of satisfaction of lower-order needs before health promotion goals can be met.

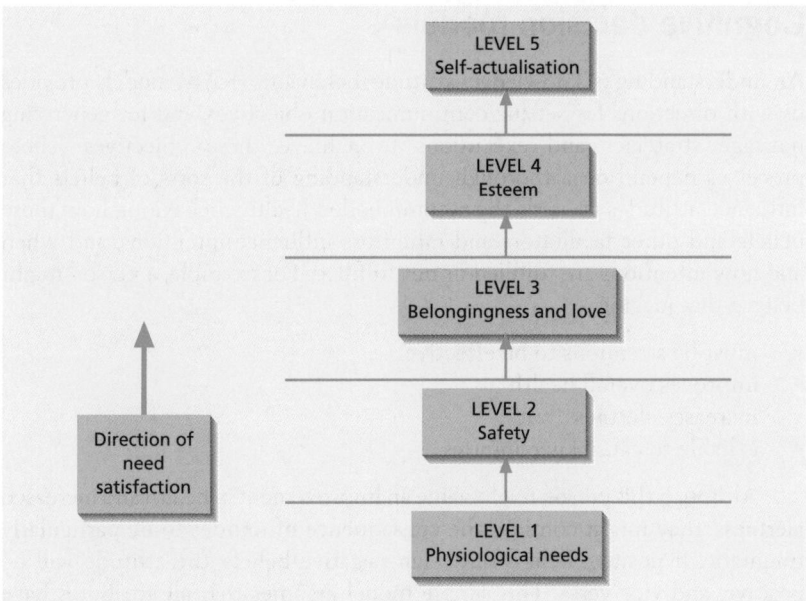

Figure 2.1: **Maslow's hierarchy of needs**   Maslow 1968

Models of behaviour change

There are numerous models of behaviour change, from individual to organisational to system perspectives. Darnton (2008) identified some 60 models, with approximately half of those having some presence in the literature. Not unexpectedly, there is considerable overlap between many models.

A useful binary classification of such models is that some (the vast majority) emphasise how beliefs and attitudes influence individual decision making and behaviour change, while others emphasise how behaviour change occurs over time for individuals or populations (Donovan 2011; Donovan & Henley 2010). The former are generally known as 'cognitive decision models' or knowledge–attitude–behaviour models; the latter are known as stages of change models when referring to changes in individuals' beliefs and attitudes over time, and as diffusion models when relating to how ideas and behaviours are adopted and spread throughout a community or population. We first describe cognitive decision models and include a brief discussion of two concepts generally absent from these models: morality and legitimacy. Applied behaviour analysis principles are also included to further emphasise that we must translate people's beliefs, attitudes and intentions into action, and that to do this, we must be aware of the necessary environmental factors and skills that will facilitate this translation.

33

Cognitive decision models

An understanding of knowledge–attitude–behaviour (KAB) models provides us with directions for setting communication objectives, and for generating message strategies and executions to achieve these objectives. These processes depend on a thorough understanding of the sorts of beliefs that influence attitudes towards the recommended healthy behaviour, how these beliefs and other facilitators and inhibitors influence intentions, and when and how intentions are fulfilled or not fulfilled. For example, a person might believe that jogging:

- must be strenuous to be effective
- improves overall health
- increases alertness, but
- is liable to cause knee injuries.

Although this person might value an improvement in health and increased alertness, they might consider the consequence of injuries to be particularly traumatic. If positive beliefs outweigh negative beliefs, the attitude will be positive, and vice versa. This simple model assumes that all attributes have equal weighting. But this is generally not so. In the above example, a person with a knee injury might place far greater importance on this attribute than on the other attributes, and far greater importance on it than individuals who do not have any prior knee problems. That is, different individuals might have different importance ratings for the same attribute.

Below, we describe several of the major models used in health promotion and the ways in which these have attempted to get around these problems. Most of these models are based on the assumption that an individual's beliefs about a person, group, issue, object or behaviour will determine the individual's attitude with respect to that person, group, issue, object or behaviour. Subject to social norms and self-efficacy, these attitudes in turn predict how the individual intends to act with regard to that person, group, issue, object or behaviour. Finally, whether or not these intentions result in behaviour will depend on environmental facilitators and inhibitors, both perceived and actual, and both situational (temporary) and structural (enduring). In short, for example, favourable attitudes and intentions towards purchasing and consuming more fruit and vegetables will only translate into behaviour where good quality fruit and vegetables are readily available at a competitive price.

The KAB or 'social-cognition' models conceptualise the influences on behaviour, and hence provide a framework for formative research, strategy development and campaign evaluation. In general, changes in the major components in these models, such as attitudes, norms and efficacy, have been found to be good predictors of changes in behaviours and intentions (Webb & Sheeran 2006).

The cognitive dissonance model

There have been several attitude theories based on the notion that people seek internal consistency between their beliefs, attitudes and behaviour, and that inconsistency is a psychologically uncomfortable state that leads to efforts to avoid or eliminate inconsistencies. The most influential of these theories has been that of Festinger's (1957) cognitive dissonance theory (CDT). CDT is concerned with the nature of the relations between various beliefs or 'cognitions'. Beliefs or cognitions might be:

- unrelated, or
- consistent (consonant), or
- inconsistent (dissonant: i.e. in conflict).

For example, a belief that sexually transmitted chlamydial infection is a common disease, together with an intention to insist on condom use, are consonant beliefs, whereas a belief that smoking causes cancer, together with an intention to continue smoking, are dissonant beliefs. The theory states that people will attempt to avoid dissonant experiences and that people experiencing dissonance will attempt to reduce it by changing their beliefs in a consonant direction. Efforts to reduce the dissonance will vary according to the degree of dissonance experienced. Mild dissonance might be ignored. The degree of dissonance will depend on the importance of the dissonance issue and the degree of disparity between the sets of dissonant cognitions; that is, dissonance is rarely experienced between just two cognitions, but rather between two sets of cognitions. As noted earlier, people generally hold a number of both negative and positive beliefs about health issues. A young smoker who believes that smoking is sophisticated, reduces anxiety and provides self-confidence in social situations, yet is harmful to health, smelly and expensive, might experience little dissonance because these two sets are relatively balanced. However, if cost has a greater degree of importance than the perceived benefits, then there will be a greater degree of dissonance.

Dissonance can be reduced in a number of ways:

- by adding new beliefs, or
- by altering beliefs, or
- by altering the importance of the beliefs or the importance of the issue per se.

For example, adding beliefs that cigarette smoke contains toxic chemicals and that research by cigarette companies themselves confirms a link between smoking and cancer could move the above smoker into a dissonant state—resulting in attempts to quit to reduce the dissonance. Reducing the perceived likelihood of contracting a sexually transmitted disease will reduce the dissonance associated with a failure to use condoms. People who do not participate in physical activity, and who experience dissonance, might decide that the issue of exercise is simply not that important, and that other aspects of health—such as diet and relaxation—are far more important.

Many attempts to reduce dissonance are similar to what are termed cognitive defence mechanisms, or rationalisations. Credible sources such as celebrities or experts are sometimes used to create dissonance by having a trusted source (e.g. a popular footballer) deliver a message (smoking is 'uncool') that the target audience (young smokers) has previously rejected. The target is then faced with rejecting the trusted source, with accepting the previously rejected message, or with rationalising that the source is insincere in this regard ('he's being paid to say that!'). Another possible outcome is that the message is partly accepted and the source is simultaneously downgraded.

Dissonance theory also helps us understand selective attention and perception: avoiding messages that are inconsistent with one's beliefs avoids the uncomfortable state of dissonance, as does reinterpreting dissonant information in a way that is consonant with one's cognitions. Overall, the dissonance model helps to explain why people act in ways that are often regarded as irrational and inconsistent.

The health belief model

The health belief model (Rosenstock 1974) (see Figure 2.2) is one of the oldest attempts to explain health behaviour. It was developed from work carried out in the 1950s, largely influenced by the works of the social psychologist Kurt Lewin. The principal tenets of the model are the way in which individuals perceive the world and how these perceptions motivate their behaviour. The model postulates that the readiness to take action for health stems from an individual's perception of his or her susceptibility to disease, its potential severity and the availability of an effective method for averting the disease. For example, mothers will insist on immunisation if they believe their child could contract a disease, that the disease could have severe consequences and that immunisation could eliminate the danger. Health-related action, then, is thought to depend on the simultaneous occurrence of three issues:

- whether the health issue is relevant
- whether the threat from it is regarded as important
- whether it's thought that doing something about it would reduce the threat.

More recently, the health belief model has been expanded to include the notion of 'self-efficacy': the belief that one has the ability to implement any change. Overall, then, for a behavioural change to succeed, individuals must have the incentive to change, feel threatened by their current behaviour, feel competent to implement a change and feel that a change will be beneficial at an acceptable cost.

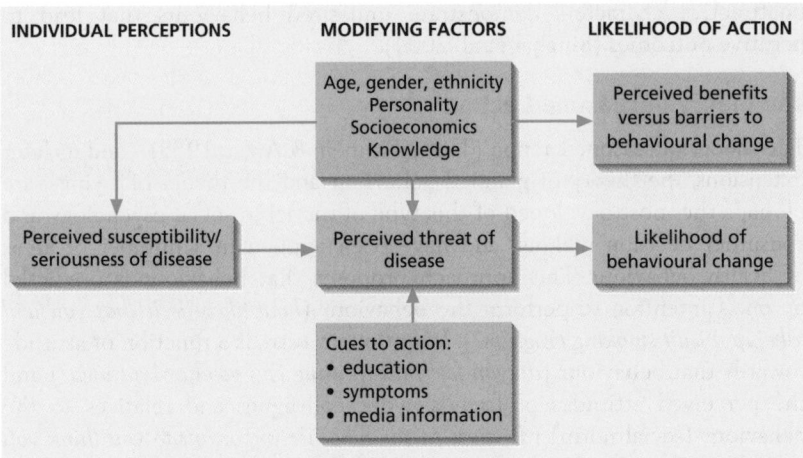

INDIVIDUAL PERCEPTIONS   MODIFYING FACTORS   LIKELIHOOD OF ACTION

Age, gender, ethnicity
Personality
Socioeconomics
Knowledge

Perceived benefits
versus barriers to
behavioural change

Perceived susceptibility/
seriousness of disease

Perceived threat of
disease

Likelihood of
behavioural change

Cues to action:
• education
• symptoms
• media information

Figure 2.2: **The health belief model**   Adapted from Rosenstock 1974

The social learning theory model

Social learning theory was developed by Bandura (1977) and was perhaps the first theory of this type to introduce the notion of self-efficacy. Social learning theory is based on the belief that behaviour is determined by expectancies and incentives, in particular by expectancies about:

- environmental cues (i.e. beliefs about how events are linked and what leads to what)
- consequences of one's actions (i.e. how the behaviour is likely to influence outcomes)
- competency to perform the behaviour needed to influence outcomes (i.e. self-efficacy).

An incentive is defined as the value of a particular object or outcome. This might be health status, better looks or feeling better. Hence, for example, people who value changing their lifestyles to healthier behaviour will do so if they believe that:

- their current lifestyle poses a threat to any valued outcome (e.g. health or appearance)
- changes will reduce the threats, whether physical or psychological
- they are personally capable of adopting the new behaviour.

The social learning theory model forms the basis for 'edutainment': the inclusion of pro-health and pro-social messages in entertainment vehicles such as soap operas. In these soap operas, desired behaviours are modelled by admirable characters and are shown to lead to positive outcomes, while unattractive characters demonstrate undesired behaviours that lead to negative outcomes (Singhal et al. 2004).

The theory of reasoned action

The theory of reasoned action (TRA)(Fishbein & Ajzen 1975)—and its later extensions, the theory of planned behaviour and the theory of trying—are perhaps the most developed of this type of model in social psychology and consumer decision making, and have been applied in a number of areas of health behaviour. This approach proposes that behaviour is predicted by one's intention to perform the behaviour (*how likely is it that you will take up a quit smoking program?*). Intention, in turn, is a function of attitude towards that behaviour (*do you feel that quitting is a good or bad idea?*) and the perceived attitudes of friends, work colleagues and relatives to the behaviour (social norm) (*do most people who are important to you think you should quit?*). Attitude is a function of beliefs about the consequences of the behaviour (*what are the outcomes of quitting?*) weighted by an evaluation of the importance of each outcome (*how important are these outcomes to you?*). Social norm is a function of expectations of significant others (*does your spouse or a close friend think that you should quit?*) weighted by the motivation to conform with each significant other (*how important is it to do what your spouse, or that friend wants?*).

The Fishbein and Ajzen model (Figure 2.3) has two important features. First, there is a clear distinction between:

- attitudes towards objects, issues, events per se
- attitudes towards behaving in a certain way towards these objects, issues and events.

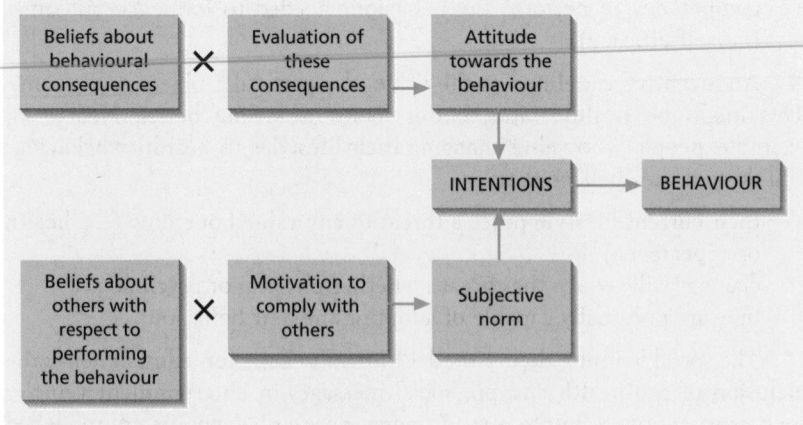

Figure 2.3: Theory of reasoned action

For example, an individual might have a favourable attitude towards Mercedes-Benz cars but a negative attitude towards actually buying one because this would involve borrowing a substantial amount of money at a high interest rate. Similarly, an individual might have a favourable attitude towards condoms per se but a negative attitude towards actually buying or carrying condoms. Hence, when exploring beliefs and attitudes to predict intentions and behaviour, it is necessary to be precise in terms of whether we are measuring attitudes towards an issue per se (e.g. exercise) or attitudes towards engaging in a certain form of behaviour (e.g. exercising). Furthermore, to predict intentions accurately, it is necessary to ensure that all relevant beliefs are uncovered. For example, it might be found that attitudes towards using condoms are favourable because only beliefs that were evaluated positively were included and beliefs that were evaluated negatively were unintentionally omitted. Formative (usually qualitative) research—based on group discussions or individual depth interviews—is usually necessary to ensure that we are aware of all relevant beliefs that could contribute to an individual's overall attitude—and hence intentions.

Fishbein and Ajzen (1975) also distinguish between:

- the individual's beliefs related to the object or issues per se
- the individual's beliefs about what other people think about the issue— and how others think they should behave towards the issue (known as normative beliefs).

Hence, the Fishbein model incorporates social norms as an influence on attitudes and behaviour. For example, an individual's attitude towards switching from a normal-strength beer to a reduced-alcohol beer will be a function of two components:

- his or her beliefs about the consequences of the behaviour (e.g. fewer hangovers, increased alertness, less risk of exceeding 0.05 per cent if breath tested, less full-bodied taste), weighted by an evaluation of the beliefs (how positively or negatively the consequences—such as fewer hangovers, increased alertness and less taste—are viewed)
- normative beliefs about how relevant others (i.e. friends, workmates and family) would view this form of behaviour (e.g. approve or disapprove), weighted by how important each of these relevant others is to the individual (e.g. workmates' opinions might be far more important than a spouse's opinion, or vice versa).

Again, it is necessary to ensure that all relevant beliefs of individuals, groups and populations are included in any measure of normative beliefs.

Fishbein and Ajzen's model has spawned a number of extensions, most notably the theory of planned behaviour (TPB) (Ajzen 1988) and the theory of trying (TT) (Bagozzi & Warshaw 1990). The theory of planned behaviour

(Ajzen 1988) added a further component influencing intentions: the extent to which the individual perceives the behaviour to be under voluntary control, which is a function of perceived individual capabilities and environmental restrictions or facilitators. Thus, even where attitudes are positive and social norms are supportive, if someone believes adoption of a recommended form of behaviour is beyond their control, they are unlikely to do it.

Both the TRA and TPB have been used quite extensively across a number of consumer-purchasing, lifestyle and health behaviours (particularly smoking, exercise and STI prevention), with generally good results for all of the major variables in the models in terms of predicting intentions or behaviours (Donovan & Henley 2010). For example, the '1% or Less' milk campaign in Wheeling, West Virginia, was based on the TRA and the compatibility principle. It resulted in a significant increase in low-fat milk share (29% to 46%) with 34 per cent of a Wheeling sample reporting switching versus 4 per cent of a comparison community. Analysis of the data showed that the intervention increased intention and attitude (but not subjective norm), and there were significant increases in beliefs about the healthiness, taste and cost of low-fat milk (Booth-Butterfield & Reger 2004). More recent research has provided support for the usefulness of the TPB in predicting adolescent athletes' intentions to use doping substances (Lucidi et al. 2008).

The theory of trying

Building on Fishbein's theory of reasoned action in the field of consumer research, Bagozzi and Warshaw's (1990) TT has two major elements of interest:

*   It focuses on the individual's goals and separates trying to achieve these goals (i.e. attempting to quit smoking) from actual attainment of the goals (i.e. successfully quitting smoking). This is a far more realistic focus. For example, rather than attempting to determine the predictors of successful quitting, we should first determine the predictors of *trying* to quit.
*   It introduces people's beliefs about the process of trying to adopt a recommended behaviour and their attitudes towards success and failure. These are covered to some extent by other models in terms of perceived costs involved in adopting a recommended behaviour, but are conceptually clearer in TT.

Figure 2.4 shows that an individual's overall attitude towards trying to adopt some behaviour (e.g. reducing fat intake) to reach a goal (e.g. losing weight) is a function of three factors:

*   the individual's attitude towards succeeding and perceived expectation of success
*   the individual's attitude towards failing and perceived expectation of failing
*   the individual's attitude towards the process of trying to lose weight.

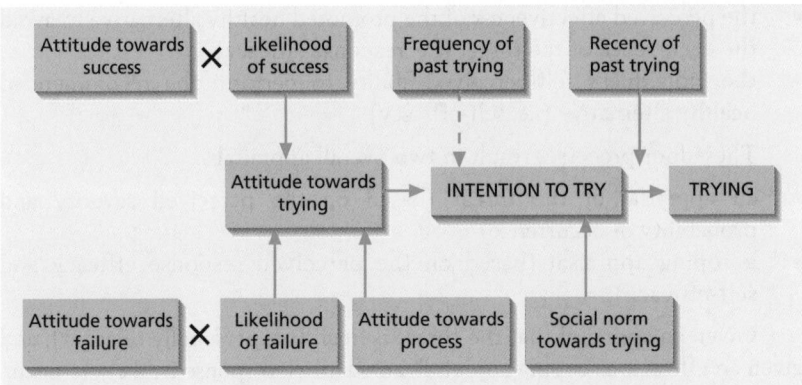

Figure 2.4: **Theory of trying**   Adapted from Bagozzi and Warshaw 1990

Again, all of the above attitudes are based on various beliefs about consequences. These include beliefs about the consequences of successfully losing weight (e.g. feeling healthier), beliefs about the consequences of not losing weight (e.g. feeling depressed), beliefs about the process of actually losing weight (e.g. feeling hungry often), and the evaluation of each of these consequences. An individual's intention to try to lose weight, then, will be determined by:

- their overall attitude towards trying to lose weight
- social norms about trying to lose weight (i.e. beliefs about relevant others' attitudes towards the individual losing weight)
- the number of times the individual has tried to lose weight before.

Finally, actually trying to lose weight will be determined by:

- the individual's intention to try to lose weight
- the time since the last trial.

Protection motivation theory

Protection motivation theory (PMT) was developed by Rogers (1975), originally as a model of fear arousal to explain the motivational effect of fear or anxiety resulting from 'threat' communications. The theory assumes that people are motivated to protect themselves not only from physical threats but also from social and psychological threats (Rogers 1975, 1983). PMT postulates four mental processes that appraise the presented health information, or threat, and that mediate attitudinal and behavioural change:

- the perceived severity of the threatened harmful event
- the perceived likelihood that the threatened outcome will occur (i.e. perceived vulnerability)

- the perceived effectiveness of the promoted healthy alternative to avoid the occurrence of the threat (i.e. response efficacy)
- the individual's self-perceived ability to perform the recommended healthy alternative (i.e. self-efficacy).

These four processes result in two overall appraisals:

- an appraisal of the threat (based on the perceived severity and probability of occurrence)
- a coping appraisal (based on the perceived response efficacy and self-efficacy).

Given an appraisal that the threat is 'real' (i.e. personally relevant), and given an efficacious coping appraisal, an adaptive response is likely to occur. If the threat appraisal is discounted (e.g. by various defence mechanisms or rationalisations, such as 'it won't happen to me'), or the recommended alternative behaviour is not seen to be viable or effective (e.g. older smokers telling themselves the 'damage is already done' and hence 'quitting now won't help'), a maladaptive response is likely to occur (i.e. continuing to smoke or even increasing smoking).

Rogers later added two further factors: response costs (perceived and actual) that inhibit adoption of the desired behaviour, and perceived rewards of continuing the undesirable behaviour that facilitate its continuation.

PMT has been applied in a number of health areas, including exercise, alcohol consumption, smoking, breast cancer screening and STIs, predicting intentions to engage in antinuclear war behaviours, earthquake preparedness

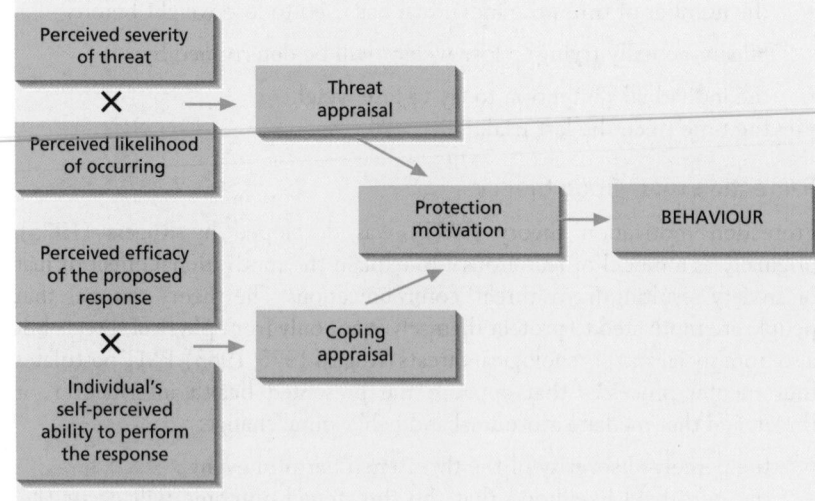

Figure 2.5: **Protection motivation theory**

and burglary prevention (Donovan 2011; Donovan & Henley 2010). In general, the concepts of vulnerability and coping appraisal—particularly self-efficacy—have been found to be significant predictors of intention and behaviour change. For example, a University of Utrecht study in the Netherlands of obese subjects in a weight-loss program found that those who at the start perceived themselves better able to control their weight and eating behaviour lost significantly more weight than the others. Strong self-efficacy was in fact the best predictor of weight-loss success (Squires 2005). The implication is that such interventions must include ways of building people's perceived (and actual) self-efficacy.

The PMT model emphasises the appraisal of threatening or supposedly fear-arousing communications. In its present form it does not allow for the assessment of messages that emphasise the positive effects or benefits of adopting the recommended behaviour. For example, both the positive benefits of exercising (e.g. enjoyment, social approval, mastery, alertness) and the avoidance of disadvantages by exercising (e.g. avoidance of heart disease) can be presented together, and often are (Donovan & Francas 1990). Hence, a more comprehensive model would include additional mediating processes of the perceived attractiveness of the positive benefits to be gained by adopting the recommended behaviour, and the perceived efficacy of that behaviour to deliver those benefits.

Behaviour modification—applied behavioural analysis

Many public health and injury prevention programs are aimed at ceasing or decreasing undesired behaviours (e.g. don't drink and drive, don't exceed the speed limit, reduce speed, eat less fat, quit smoking, reduce alcohol consumption), while others are aimed at adopting or increasing desired behaviours (e.g. drink reduced-alcohol beer in preference to full-strength beer, use a condom, eat more fruit and vegetables, walk to the bus stop/ up the stairs/to the shop). The question in many situations therefore is whether the emphasis should be on increasing the desired behaviour or on decreasing the undesired behaviour. For example, for targeting reduced obesity in children, should we focus on reducing the time spent watching TV and playing video games (i.e. reduce inactivity) or focus on increasing the children's level of physical activity? Regardless of the answer, learning theory draws our attention to the fact that different strategies might be more appropriate for decreasing or ceasing a particular behaviour versus increasing or adopting a behaviour. This has significant implications for message strategies in communication materials and for direct behavioural interventions.

Table 2.1: Behaviour modification strategies

Procedure following behaviour:		
Consequence type	Deliver consequence	Remove consequence
Good/pleasant	Positive reinforcement (increases response)	Negative punishment (decreases response)
Bad/unpleasant	Positive punishment (decreases response)	Negative reinforcement (increases response)

Behaviour modification (the terms 'behaviour modification' and 'applied behaviour analysis' are generally interchangeable) is defined as the systematic application of principles derived from learning theory to altering environment–behaviour relationships in order to strengthen adaptive behaviours and weaken maladaptive behaviours (Elder et al. 1994). Behaviour modification is based on the assumption that behaviour is determined by environmental antecedents and consequences (Elder et al. 1994; Geller 1989).

Table 2.1 delineates two ways of *increasing* a behaviour and two ways of *decreasing* a behaviour. The former are termed *reinforcement* strategies, whereas the latter are termed *punishment* strategies. Table 2.1 is an elaboration of the simple principle that a behaviour followed by a positive outcome will tend to be repeated whereas a behaviour that attracts a negative outcome will tend to cease. In Table 2.1, the impact on a behaviour is shown to be a function of two binary dimensions: (a) whether the behaviour results in the *removal* or *delivery* of a consequence; and (b) whether that consequence is a *positive* or *negative* outcome.

Table 2.1 shows that the two ways of increasing or reinforcing a behaviour are:

- *Positive reinforcement*—the behaviour is followed by a pleasant consequence (e.g. group socialising after exercise).
- *Negative reinforcement*—the behaviour is followed by removal of an unpleasant situation (e.g. headache and tension gone after meditation).

The two ways of decreasing or punishing a behaviour are:

- *Positive punishment*—the behaviour is followed by an unpleasant consequence (e.g. speeding is followed by a fine).
- *Negative punishment* (or 'response cost')—the behaviour is followed by removal of a pleasant situation (e.g. drunk driving is followed by a loss of licence and subsequent limitations on mobility and socialising).

Two other processes are also relevant:

- *Extinction*—a behaviour will decrease and eventually cease (extinguish) if previously applied positive consequences are discontinued or barriers prevent them being obtained. For example, walking may decrease if aesthetic features of the environment are removed or friends are no longer available to walk with; blood donating behaviour will decline if donors have to visit a central location rather than being able to donate at the worksite.

* *Response facilitation*—a behaviour will strengthen or re-emerge if a punishment is discontinued. For example, an athlete may revert to using performance enhancing drugs when the level of random testing is reduced; speeding behaviour returns after speed camera use declines.

In designing interventions, formative research is necessary to determine the appropriate reinforcers and punishments for the various target groups. Some people may be motivated primarily by social recognition rewards, others by financial incentives, and others by gifts. Young males fear the loss of their driving licence more than the threat of physical harm to themselves, and the GutBusters® program for men emphasised the 'looking good' benefit of weight loss and increased physical activity rather than health benefits.

Feedback on positive results, such as number of accident-free days in a workplace, is an important reinforcer. Health promotion advocates should remember that as well as writing to politicians and policy makers whom they wish to persuade, they should also write to those already on side, with reinforcing messages thanking them for their support. Another lesson from behaviour modification is to identify the reinforcers of the behaviours we wish to reduce or eliminate. Such an understanding is liable to lead to more sustained change if attempts are then made to either substitute benign reinforcers or take away the need for the reinforcers in the first place. For example, much alcohol and drug abuse is related to escaping from reality. Hence interventions making reality more tolerable, or indeed enjoyable, are required.

Conditional cash incentives to the poor, in several countries, have resulted in positive health outcomes—especially for children. Kane and colleagues (2004) analysed 47 trials of cash incentives for preventive health behaviours such as immunisation, cancer screening, condom purchase, education session attendance, prenatal care, weight loss and tuberculosis screening. They found that these incentives were generally successful in that they worked for around 73 per cent of the cases studied. However, there are some ethical and sustainability issues around offering financial incentives, and there are clearly problems in determining how much the incentive should be and for how long it should be paid.

Most of the above deals with the behaviour–consequence link. Interventions can also facilitate the desired behavioural response by looking at the antecedent–behaviour link:

* Environments should be designed to make the behaviour change easy, such as worksite exercise rooms and showers or smaller plates in restaurants to limit food portions.

- Reminder signs can be very effective. A 'take the stairs' sign placed near an elevator increased use of the stairs dramatically, 'belt up' signs at car park exits increase seat belt use and nutrition information on menus increases healthy food selections.
- Opinion leaders, experts and celebrities can be used to demonstrate the behaviour or wear clothing promoting the behaviour.
- Target individuals can be encouraged to make public commitments to adopt the desired behaviour.
- Educational materials with behavioural tips are also useful; quitting smokers are encouraged to identify environmental cues that trigger smoking and to remove them.
- Education sessions should include interactive demonstrations rather than just passive lecturing ('tell them and they'll forget—demonstrate and they'll remember—involve them and they'll understand').

Much of the above can be termed 'choice architecture', introduced in the book *Nudge* (Thaler & Sunstein 2008). The premise of the book is that the environment can be designed to reduce opportunities for 'bad' choices and to 'nudge' people into desirable choices while retaining 'freedom of choice'. While this concept is hardly novel, the book reminds us that we can extend these ideas into better decision making in neglected economic areas such as savings plans, insurance and retirement planning decisions.

Morality and legitimacy

Morality refers to an individual's beliefs about whether certain actions are 'right or wrong', or whether they 'should or should not' take that action. Legitimacy refers to an individual's beliefs about whether laws are justified, whether these laws are applied equally, and whether punishments for transgressions are fair (Tyler 1990, 1997). The concept of legitimacy applies not only to judicial legislation but also to organisations' rules, regulations and policies. In general, people are more likely to obey rules that they believe are justified and that are enforced in a fair and unbiased manner.

With some reflection, and given the use of 'laws' to regulate and influence behaviour, both concepts clearly have considerable relevance in some areas of health promotion and injury prevention. However, they have been largely neglected in social change models, and particularly in public health research and intervention strategies. This neglect is surprising given the historical links between health and (religious) morality (Thomas 1997), and the fact that Fishbein's theory of reasoned action originally included the concept of moral or personal norms. Triandis's (1977) model included personal normative beliefs, but his model has attracted limited attention in health and social interventions.

Legislation is widely used to regulate a broad range of activities such as driving behaviours, underage alcohol and tobacco consumption, drug use, land degradation and toxic waste disposal, lighting fires in forests, littering behaviour, physical abuse, child abuse and neglect, and so on. Hence it is important to assess people's perceived legitimacy of the laws and the authorities behind the laws in these areas. In fact, crime prevention is one area where public health and antiviolence professionals are beginning to come together (WHO 2002), and some social marketers are also taking an interest (e.g. Hastings, Stead & MacFadyen 2002). Criminologists have been developing conceptual frameworks in these areas, with striking similarities to concepts in cognitive decision models as described in this chapter (e.g. Vila 1994).

Norman and Connor (1996) found only a few studies that incorporated measures of moral norms within the public health domain. Such studies include explaining altruism and helping behaviour such as donating blood and intentions to donate organs. Other studies have found measures of moral norms to be predictive of recycling behaviour, eating genetically produced food, buying milk, using condoms and committing driving violations (see Donovan & Henley 2010). However, other than road safety, few public health and public policy campaigns have considered the use of moral or legitimacy appeals. Road safety campaigns have emphasised that drinking and driving is a danger to others and hence morally unacceptable. Legitimacy has also been part of road safety campaigns. For example, 'Buckle Up. It's the Law' in the US appeals directly to compliance because it is a legal requirement, while the UK's 'It's 30 for A Reason' can be seen as an attempt to increase people's perceived justification (legitimacy) for that speed limit in built-up areas.

An interesting study in light of 'situational prompts' noted elsewhere in this chapter is that of Shu and colleagues' (2009) studies of choices in ethical-dilemma-type scenarios where subjects had the opportunity to carry out an unethical behaviour undetected. They found that many people almost unthinkingly chose the unethical behaviour. However, they also found that increasing moral salience by simply having people read or sign an honour code significantly reduced or eliminated unethical behaviour.

Moral disengagement

According to Bandura (2002), individuals refrain from behaving in ways that breach their moral codes because of self-condemnation. However, such self-regulation is subject to social and situational influences and individuals may succumb to behaviours that transgress their moral codes in various situations. In these cases, the individual then 'rationalises' the transgression via various mechanisms that excuse or justify the behaviour. This is known as 'moral disengagement', and, along with self-regulatory efficacy, is beginning to be used to explain young people's alcohol, tobacco and drug use (Newton, Havard & Teesson 2012) and the use of performance enhancing drugs (Boardley & Kavussanu 2007).

Change models

The transtheoretical stages of change model

This model of behaviour change derives from Prochaska's clinical work with cigarette and drug addiction (Prochaska & Di Clemente 1984, 1986). The stages of change concept not only delineates the stages an individual goes through during a behaviour change, but also is used to divide the target population (e.g. smokers, non-exercisers, coercive parents, men who use violence, drug users) into sub-segments depending on their stage in progression towards adoption of the desired behaviour (i.e. quitting smoking, taking up exercise, using positive parenting practices, ceasing violent behaviour, stopping drug use) (see Prochaska et al. 2005, 2007).

The stages are:

1. *Precontemplation*—where the individual is not considering modifying their undesired behaviour.
2. *Contemplation*—where the individual is considering changing an undesired behaviour, but not in the immediate future.
3. *Preparation*—where the individual plans to try to change the undesired behaviour in the immediate future (that is, in the next 2 weeks or an appropriate timeframe).
4. *Action*—the immediate (6-month) period following trial and adoption of the recommended behaviour and cessation of the undesired behaviour.
5. *Maintenance*—the period following the action stage until the undesired behaviour is fully extinguished.
6. *Termination*—when the problem behaviour is completely eliminated, that is, 'zero temptation across all problem situations'.

It is claimed that individuals at different stages of change would have different attitudes, beliefs and motivations with respect to the (desired) new behaviour, and hence different treatment approaches and communication strategies may be necessary for individuals in the different stages of change. There is some support for these claims over a variety of areas, but particularly smoking, nutrition and exercise (de Vet et al. 2008; Oman and King 1998; Spencer et al. 2006). Donovan and Henley (2010) report that the model has also been applied across a variety of countries and sub-groups, including the UK, African-American and Hispanic sub-populations in the US, Holland, Sweden, Spain and 15 European Union states.

Prochaska and colleagues (1994) describe nine activities or processes of change that individuals use to proceed through the stages of change:

1. *Consciousness raising*—increasing awareness about the problem.
2. *Emotional arousal*—dramatic expressions of the problem and consequences.

3. *Self re-evaluation*—reappraisal of the problem and its inconsistency with self-values.
4. *Commitment*—choosing to change and making a public commitment to do so.
5. *Social liberation*—choosing social environments that foster or facilitate change.
6. *Relationship fostering*—getting help from others, professional or otherwise.
7. *Counter-conditioning*—substituting alternatives.
8. *Reward*—administering self-praise or other positive experiences for dealing with the problem.
9. *Environmental control*—restructuring of the environment to reduce temptations and opportunities.

The processes at the top of the list are experiential, whereas those lower in the list are behavioural. The former occur more in the earlier stages of change, the latter in the later stages. The transtheoretical model also incorporates the notion of decisional balance: that an evaluation of the costs (cons) and benefits (pros) of making the change varies over the stages, with cons outweighing pros in precontemplation, pros outweighing cons in the action stage, with crossing over occurring during contemplation.

Donovan and colleagues (1999) tested three anti-smoking ads and analysed the results for precontemplators, contemplators and those in the ready-for-action and action stages. Figure 2.6 shows a significant relationship between the stages of change and the ads' impact on intentions to quit or cut

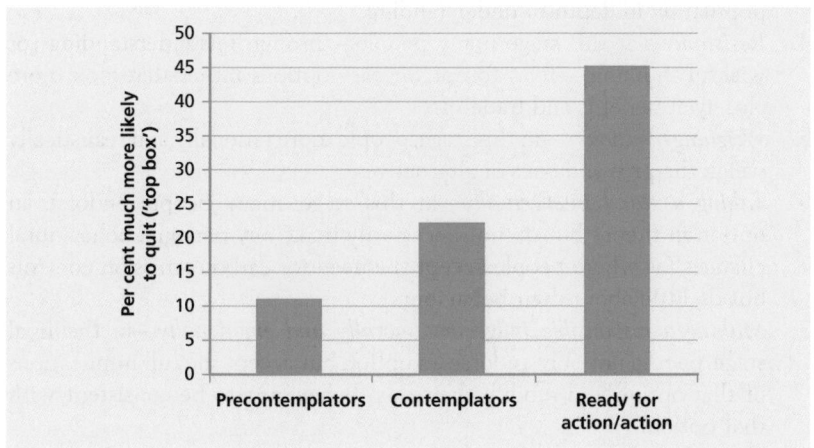

Figure 2.6: Impact of Quit ads on likelihood of quitting or cutting down by smokers' stage of change   Donovan et al. 1999

down the amount smoked. These results confirm that smokers in the different stages of change react quite differently to anti-smoking communications.

The stages of change concept is widely used but perhaps not always properly understood, especially with regard to the various processes applicable to each of the stages (Whitelaw et al. 1999). Nevertheless, regardless of whether one adopts Prochaska's recommended intervention processes for the various stages, the model is very useful as a segmentation method for recruiting sub-samples for formative research and for targeting in those areas most related to addictive behaviours, from whence it was derived. Further, regardless of the finer points of these models, the concept of 'readiness to change' is a useful one in a practical sense. The Western Australian 'Freedom from Fear' domestic violence campaign targets 'men who are aware of their problem with violence and want to change'. In stages terminology that means violent men in the contemplator and ready for action stages (Donovan et al. 2000). In fact the booklet for men explicitly states on the cover: 'For men who want to change'.

Stages of change for public opinion

At a broader level, the much respected public opinion tracker Daniel Yankelovich (1992) has delineated seven stages of public opinion change. Yankelovich's seven stages are:

1. *Dawning awareness*—this is when people first begin to become aware of an issue, usually through mass media news reports.
2. *A sense of urgency*—people move from simple awareness of an issue to developing a sense of urgency about needing to form an opinion about it.
3. *Discovering the choices*—people start to explore choices and look at the pros and cons of the issue, although there is widespread variation in the population in depth of understanding.
4. *Resistance*—at this stage many people—through misunderstanding (or wishful thinking)—tend to opt for easy options rather that look more closely at benefits and trade-offs.
5. *Weighing the choices*—in this stage, people more rationally and realistically weigh the pros and cons of alternatives.
6. *Taking a stand intellectually*—at this stage, many people endorse an option in theory but do not necessarily make any personal behavioural changes (as where people accept the need for carbon emission controls but do little about their behaviours).
7. *Making a responsible judgement morally and emotionally*—in the final stage, people not only endorse an option but accept the full implications of that option and modify their own behaviours to be consistent with that option.

Yankelovich's model is particularly useful for those planning advocacy campaigns based on mobilising public opinion.

Community readiness model

Another useful model, particularly for community-based interventions in developing countries or remote/rural communities in developed countries, is the community readiness model (Kelly et al. 2003). This model—as its name suggests—is concerned with the stages a community must go through to be ready for an intervention, rather than the stages of progression after an intervention occurs. The model first looks at factors such as the community's current knowledge, actions and attitudes towards the issue in question, leadership in the community and community resources. It then delineates nine stages, from 'no awareness' through various stages of denial, preplanning, preparation and training, through to implementation of the intervention with a 'high level of community ownership'.

Diffusion theory

Everett Rogers first published his book *Diffusion of Innovations* in 1962. The concept has been readily adopted in commercial marketing (to predict new product adoption) and is widely used to explain the adoption of public health and agricultural processes in particular in developing countries. However, it is only in the past 15 years or so that it has attracted much attention in the public health area in developed countries. The general concept no doubt also received an impetus from Gladwell's (2000) book *The Tipping Point*.

Rogers (1995) defines 'diffusion' as the process by which an innovation is communicated through certain channels over time among the members of a social system. Diffusion theory applies to both planned and unplanned diffusions, and to both desirable and undesirable innovations (e.g. the rapid adoption of the cocaine variant 'crack' in the US). Figure 2.7 shows the rate of diffusion of three innovations.

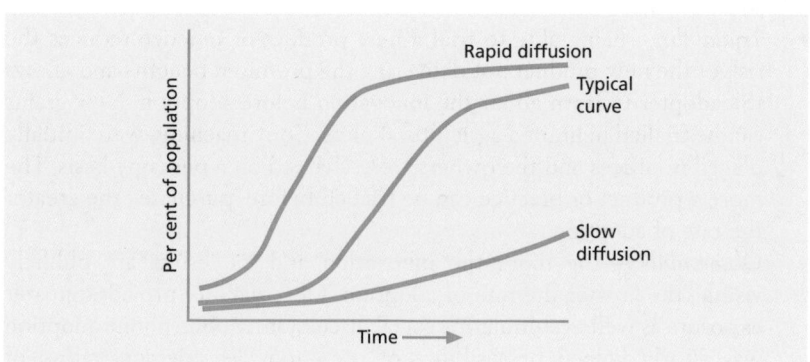

Figure 2.7: **Diffusion of innovations**

Many innovations 'take off' at about the 20 per cent adoption mark, when, according to Rogers (1995), interpersonal networks become activated so that a critical mass of adopters begins using an innovation.

From the health promotion practitioner's point of view, one of the major issues is how the rate of adoption of the new idea, product or behaviour can be accelerated. This can be assessed via an analysis of each of the four main elements in diffusion: the innovation, communication channels, time, and social system.

The innovation

An innovation is an idea, product or practice that is perceived as new by the adopting population; that is, it need not be objectively 'new'. The attributes of the innovation that influence its rate of adoption are:

- *Relative advantage*—if the new product or practice is seen to be clearly 'better' than the old, then it will be adopted more readily. Relative advantage can be assessed in a variety of ways, including convenience, economy, prestige and time: email is much faster than postal mail; automated garbage trucks are perceived to be more economical than manned trucks.
- *Compatibility*—the more the new product or practice is consistent with current values and past experiences, the more readily it will be adopted. Family planning and STI prevention practices face a barrier in countries where cultural and religious values are opposed to these practices. Automated teller machines are incompatible with many people's desire for interpersonal interactions.
- *Complexity*—new practices and ideas that are easy to understand are more readily adopted than those difficult to understand or that require special skills and training. User-friendly software was a major factor in the rates of adoption of office and home computers and the new social media.
- *Trialability*—being able to trial a new product or practice reduces the risk of the new product not delivering the promised benefits and allows the adopter to learn about the innovation before adoption. New grains can be trialled in limited agricultural plots. Copy machines were initially placed in offices and the owners were charged on a per-copy basis. The more a product or practice can be trialled before 'purchase', the greater the rate of adoption.
- *Observability*—the more the innovation and its results are publicly visible, the greater the rate of adoption. Observability provides greater exposure as well as stimulating social discussion. Mobile phone adoption was clearly helped by visibility of use—and clear demonstration of effectiveness in communication.

Communication channels

Rogers (1995) suggests that mass media channels are the most effective way of creating awareness for a new idea, product or practice, whereas interpersonal channels are the most effective way of getting the target audience to accept and adopt the new idea. Rogers states that a major impediment to most planned social diffusions is that the change agent and the target are quite dissimilar ('heterophilus'). Tupperware's use of party hosts to sell products to their friends is a very good example of acknowledging that persuasion occurs best between people of similar interests. The importance of interpersonal networks in the diffusion process is one of the most important concepts of the diffusion process, and hence for community development interventions.

Time

Time can be noted on an individual basis in the sense of the time taken to move from awareness, through persuasion, to decision, then adoption. Some decision processes are relatively brief, while others may take several months. Time also can be considered in the sense of some people adopting the innovation soon after its introduction (early adopters), while others adopt only after the vast majority have adopted (laggards). In general, five groups are noted: innovators (the first 2–3%), early adopters (the next 10–15%), the early majority (the next 30–33%), the late majority (the next 30–33%) and the laggards (the final 17–20%). Effort expended on identifying the innovators and early adopters can result in a more efficiently planned diffusion. Finally, as shown in Figure 2.7, the rate of adoption can vary from very rapid to quite slow.

The social system

The social structure also influences the rate of adoption. Variables here include: the extent to which communication channels exist; the presence or absence of strong opinion leaders; the prevailing social norms and their variation between parts of the system; whether the adoption decision is an individual one or must involve collective decision making, or a single authority's decision; and whether adoption of the innovation has desirable and undesirable consequences, not just for the individual but for the social system as a whole. Rudd (2003) analyses how health policies diffuse through to general practice, given the nature of general practice and the attitudes and beliefs of general practitioners about their role in the health system. Social system factors appear particularly important in developing countries (McKee 1992), and, for example, in Indigenous communities in Australia.

Social ecology

The theory of social ecology in health promotion is another example of the shift from the downstream, individual-focused, lifestyle modification approach to a broader understanding of health protective factors. Stokols (1996) advocated the theory of social ecology as one of three complementary perspectives on health promotion:

- targeting the individual with behaviour change recommendations relating to lifestyle issues such as smoking, substance use, diet, exercise, and safety
- changing the environment to maximise health protective factors by creating a safe place, free from contagious disease and unhealthy levels of stress (caused by environmental factors such as pollution, racism or violence), in which healthy behaviours are actively facilitated and where people have access to health care
- social ecological analyses that attempt to understand the interplay between the environment and the individual, emphasising the interdependence of multiple environments and the contributions of many, diverse disciplines.

Thus, while the individual behaviour change approach may be concerned with persuasion theories and health communication, and the environmental change approach may consider urban planning and injury control, the social ecological approach focuses on aspects such as cultural change models of health, medical sociology, community health and public policy (Stokols 1996). The major contribution of the social ecological approach is that it provides a systems framework within which behavioural and environmental factors can be integrated, thereby eliminating the claimed 'blind spots' inherent in focusing on either the individual or the environmental approach. A typical ecological health evaluation involves different levels of analysis and multiple methodologies, from individual medical examinations to environmental assessments to epidemiological analyses.

Cohen and colleagues (2000) provide a useful framework based on ecological theory. They postulate four categories of structural factors that influence individuals' behaviours: the availability of protective or harmful consumer products (e.g. tobacco, alcohol, guns, fatty foods, condoms, fruit and vegetables); physical structures and physical characteristics of products (e.g. buildings, neighbourhood design, lighting, seat belts, childproof medicine containers); social structures and policies (e.g. strict versus lax enforcement of laws and policies, unsupervised youth, social norms); and media and cultural messages (e.g. advertising messages regarding materialism, depictions of violence, racism). Hence, with regard to firearms in the US, there is relatively easy availability, fear and perceived likelihood of crime facilitate purchasing, safety locks can make guns safer while other modifications make them more lethal, and television shows and movies suggest that guns are a good—and normative—way to resolve conflicts.

Synthesising the models

Behavioural scientists have now generally come to the following set of principles with respect to individuals performing a recommended behaviour:

- They must have formed an intention to perform the behaviour or made a (public) commitment to do so.
- There are no physical or structural environmental constraints that prevent the behaviour being performed.
- The individual has the skills and equipment necessary to perform the behaviour.
- Individuals perceive themselves to be capable of performing the behaviour.
- Individuals consider that the benefits/rewards of performing the behaviour outweigh the costs/disbenefits associated with performing the behaviour, including the rewards associated with *not* performing the behaviour (i.e. a positive attitude towards performing the behaviour).
- Social normative pressure to perform the behaviour is perceived to be greater than social normative pressure not to perform the behaviour.
- Individuals perceive the behaviour to be consistent with their self-image and internalised values (i.e. morally acceptable).
- Individuals perceive the behaviour to be consistent with their social roles.
- The individual's emotional reaction (or expectation) in performing the behaviour is more positive than negative.

Hence, if a violent man has formed a strong intention to call a helpline about his violence, if a telephone is easily accessible, and if the call can be made in private and with assured confidentiality, it is likely that the behaviour will occur. The remainder of the above variables primarily influence intention or facilitate/inhibit translating the intention into action.

Overall, it is clear that many of the above models, particularly the KAB models, contain similar concepts, but that no one model includes all relevant concepts. Therefore, a pragmatic, eclectic approach is advocated in practice, selecting concepts from each of the models depending on which are more or less applicable to the behaviour in question. For example, Donovan and Henley (2010) suggest the following questions need answering to develop appropriate interventions for an adult at risk of type 2 diabetes:

1. What is the individual's perceived likelihood of contracting diabetes, given no change in his or her current behaviour?
   - What beliefs or perceptions underlie this perceived likelihood?
   - If the perceived likelihood is unrealistically low, what sort of information, presented in what way, and by whom, might increase this likelihood?
   - What is his or her knowledge of the causes of diabetes?

2. What is the individual's perceived severity of contracting diabetes?
   - Is this realistic? If not, what sort of information, presented in what way, and by whom, might change this perception?

3. What is the individual's attitude towards adopting the recommended alternative behaviours such as a change in diet or more exercise?
   - Are some behaviours more acceptable than others? Why?
   - What are the perceived benefits of continuing the risk behaviours?
   - What are the perceived benefits and the disbenefits of the alternative behaviours?
   - What social and physical environment barriers inhibit adoption of the recommended dietary and exercise behaviours? What facilitators exist?

4. What is the individual's perceived likelihood of averting the threat if the recommended behaviours are adopted?
   - If this is low, on what beliefs is this perception based? What information might change this perception?

5. What are the individual's beliefs about his or her ability to adopt the recommended behaviours?
   - On what beliefs are these efficacy perceptions based?
   - Is skills training required?
   - What intermediate goals can be set to induce trial?

6. What appear to be the major motivations that would induce trial of the recommended behaviours?
   - Are positive benefits (e.g. feelings of wellness, increased capacity for physical activity) more motivating than negative benefits (e.g. avoidance of disease) for some individuals or groups, and vice versa for others?

7. What are the individual's main sources of information and advice for health?
   - Who are the major influencers?

8. How do the individual's social interactions—including the extended family, club memberships, employment and home-care role—influence his or her health beliefs and behaviours?

9. Does the individual exhibit any personality characteristics that might inhibit or facilitate the adoption of healthy behaviours?

10. What are the individual's perceptions of social norms with regard to the recommended behaviours?
    - Who are their relevant reference groups and these groups' relative influence?
    - Does the individual see the recommended behaviours as compatible with his or her social roles and self-image?

11. What are the individual's perceptions of the morality of non-compliance with the recommended behaviour and consistency with internalised values?

12. What knowledge do medical practitioners and other primary healthcare workers have of diabetes risk factors and what is their willingness to undertake preventive measures with patients exhibiting these risk factors?
13. What factors exist in the individual's social, economic, work and physical environment that facilitate and inhibit attendance at diabetes screening?
14. What factors exist in the individual's social, economic, work and physical environment that facilitate and inhibit healthy eating and exercise habits?
15. What knowledge of diabetes do health bureaucrats have and what are their attitudes towards allocating funds to prevention?

Concluding comments

The above questions show that the models described in this chapter apply to an individual's beliefs and attitudes about the risky or unhealthy behaviours in question, as well as to his or her beliefs and attitudes about broader environmental influences related to those behaviours. Formative research helps to determine the various beliefs and perceptions that underlie attitudes, motivation and behaviour. Strategies can then be devised to change these beliefs (e.g. increase the perceived likelihood of a disease occurring), change the evaluation of these beliefs (e.g. increase knowledge about the potential effects of this disease), or introduce new beliefs (e.g. that having this disease increases susceptibility to an even more feared problem).

The last five questions above are a reminder that these models are useful not only for developing campaigns targeting individuals to promote adoption or maintenance of desired behaviours and cessation of undesired behaviours, but also for developing advocacy campaigns targeting policy makers and legislators to introduce policies, regulations and legislation that will not only remove barriers to, but provide conditions that facilitate the adoption of, desired behaviours. For example, if a politician is shown survey evidence that her constituents are overwhelmingly in favour of reduced liquor outlet hours, if she is aware of considerable media publicity supporting such a move, if she is experienced at tabling motions at party and committee meetings, and if she is personally aware of the effects of excess alcohol consumption due to extended trading hours, then it is more likely that she will comply with an advocacy group's request to have the issue of liquor outlet trading hours included on the agenda of her party's next meeting. The key is to carry out appropriate additional research in advocacy areas to identify the beliefs, attitudes and skills relevant to political behaviours.

It has been suggested that some of these models might be more or less appropriate for different behaviours, and that this could be a fruitful area for future research. However, we recommend an eclectic approach as indicated in the above synthesis of the models. It is considered that a more fruitful area for research is not so much about which model best explains a particular phenomenon, but what concepts from all or any of the models are more or less relevant to particular phenomena. Related to that approach is that future research could also attempt to identify new (or abandoned) concepts (such as morality and legitimacy) that would enhance the predictability of attitudes and behaviours in particular domains. It is likely that monitoring the development and use of models in areas such as criminology, consumer behaviour, political science, social geography and sociology could be beneficial in this regard.

References

Ajzen, I., 1988, *Attitudes, Personality, and Behaviour*, Dorsey Press, Chicago.

Bagozzi, R.P., & Warshaw, P.R., 1990, Trying to consume, *J Consum Res* 17:127–40.

Bandura, A., 1977, *Social Learning Theory*, Prentice Hall, Englewood Cliffs, NJ.

Bandura, A., 2002, Selective moral disengagement in the exercise of moral agency, *J Moral Educ* 31:101–19.

Boardley, I. D., & Kavussanu, M, 2007. Development and validation of the Moral Disengagement in Sport Scale. *J Sport Exerc Psych* 29, 608–28.

Booth-Butterfield, S. & Reger, B., 2004, The message changes belief and the rest is theory: the '1% or less' milk campaign and reasoned action, *Prev Med*, 39(3), 581–8.

Cohen, D., Scribner, R., & Farley, T., 2000, A structural model of health behaviour: a pragmatic approach to explain and influence health behaviours at the population level, *Prev Med* 30(2):146–54.

Darnton, A., 2008, *Reference Report: An Overview of Behaviour Change Models and Their Uses*, Government Social Research, UK Government.

de Vet, E., de Nooijer, J., de Vries, N., & Brug, J, 2008, Testing the transtheoretical model for fruit intake: comparing web-based tailored stage-matched and stage-mismatched feedback, *Health Educ Res* 23(2):218–27.

Donovan, R.J., 2011, Theoretical models of behaviour change, in Hastings, G., Bryant, C., & Angus, K. (Eds), *The Sage Handbook of Social Marketing*, Sage, London.

Donovan, R J., & Francas, M., 1990, Understanding communication and motivation strategies, *Aust Health Rev* 10:103–14.

Donovan, R.J., Francas, M., Paterson, D., & Zappelli, R., 2000, Formative research for mass media-based campaigns: Western Australia's 'Freedom from Fear' campaign targeting male perpetrators of intimate partner violence, *Health Promot J Aust* 10(2):78–83.

Donovan, R.J., & Henley, N., 2010, *Social Marketing: An International Perspective*, Cambridge University Press, Cambridge.

Donovan, R.J., Leivers, S., & Hannaby, L., 1999, Smokers' responses to anti-smoking advertisements by stage of change. *Soc Mar Q*, 5(2):56–63, http://smq.sagepub.com/content/5/2/56.abstract, accessed May 2013.

Elder, J.P., Geller, E.S., Hovell, M.F., & Mayer, J.A., 1994, *Motivating Health Behaviour*, Delmar, NY.

Festinger, L.A., 1957, *A Theory of Cognitive Dissonance*, Stanford University Press, Palo Alto, Calif.

Fishbein, M., & Ajzen, I., 1975, *Beliefs, Attitudes, Intention and Behaviour: An Introduction to Theory and Research*, Addison-Wesley, Boston, Mass.

Geller, E.S., 1989, Applied behaviour analysis and social marketing: an integration for environmental preservation, *J Soc Issues* 45:17–36.

Gladwell, M., 2000, *The Tipping Point: How Little Things Can Make a Big Difference*, Little Brown & Company, London.

Hastings, G., Stead, M., & MacFadyen, L., 2002, Reducing prison numbers: does marketing hold the key?, *Criminal Justice Matters* 49(1):20–5.

Kane, R.L., Johnson, P.E., Town, R.J., & Butler, M., 2004, A structured review of the effect of economic incentives on consumers' preventive behaviour, *Am J Prev Med* 27(4):327–52.

Kelly, K.J., Edwards, W., Comello, M., Plested, B., Thurman, P., & Slater, M., 2003, The community readiness model: a complementary approach to social marketing, *Marketing Theory* 3(4):411–26.

Lucidi, F., Zelli, A., Mallia, L., Grano, C., Russo, P., & Violani, C., 2008, The social-cognitive mechanism regulating adolescents' use of doping substances, *J Sports Sci* 26:447–56.

Maslow, A.H., 1968, *Towards a Psychology of Being*, Van Nostrand, NY.

McKee, N., 1992, *Social Mobilisation and Social Marketing*, Southbound, Penang, Malaysia.

Newton, N.C., Havard, A., & Teesson, M., 2012, The association between moral disengagement, psychological distress, resistive self-regulatory efficacy and alcohol and cannabis use among adolescents in Sydney, Australia, *Addict Res Theory* 20(3):261–9

Norman, P., & Connor, M., 1996, The role of social cognition models in predicting health behaviours: future directions, in Conner, M., & Norman, P. (Eds.), *Predicting Health Behaviour*, Open University Press, Buckingham, pp. 197–225.

Nutbeam, D., & Harris, H., 2004, *Theory in a Nutshell: A Practical Guide to Health Promotion Theories* (2nd edn), McGraw-Hill, Sydney.

Oman, R.F., & King, A.C., 1998, Predicting the adoption and maintenance of exercise participation using self-efficacy and previous exercise participation rates, *Am J Health Promot* 12(3):154–61.

Prochaska, J.O., & DiClemente, C.C., 1984, *The Transtheoretical Approach: Crossing the Traditional Boundaries of Therapy*, Dow-Jones/Irwin, Illinois.

Prochaska, J.O., & DiClemente, C.C., 1986, Toward a comprehensive model of change, in Miller, W.R. and Heather, N. (Eds.), *Treating Addictive Behaviours: Processes of Change*. Plenum Press, New York.

Prochaska, J.O., Evers K.E., Prochaska J.M., Van Marter, D., & Johnson J.L, 2007, Efficacy and effectiveness trials: examples from smoking cessation and bullying prevention, *J Health Psychol* 12(1):170–8.

Prochaska, J.O., Norcross, J.C., & DiClemente, C.C., 1994, *Changing for Good*, Avon Books, New York.

Prochaska, J.O., Velicer, W.F., Redding, C., Rossi, J.S., Goldstein, M., DePue, J., Greene, G, W., Rossi S.R., Sun, X., Fava, J.L., Laforge, R., Rakowski, W., & Plummer, B.A., 2005, Stage-based expert systems to guide a population of primary care patients to quit smoking, eat healthier, prevent skin cancer, and receive regular mammograms, *Prev Med* 41:406–16.

Rogers, E.M., 1995, *Diffusion of Innovations* (4th edn), The Free Press, New York.

Rogers, R.W., 1975, A protection motivation theory of fear appeals and attitude change, *J Psychol* 91:93–114.

Rogers, R.W., 1983, Cognitive and physiological process in fear appeals and attitude change: a revised theory of protection motivation, in Cacioppo, J., & Petty, R. (Eds), *Social Psychophysiology*, Guilford Press, New York.

Rosenstock, I.M., 1974, Historical models of the health belief model, in Becker, M.H. (Ed.), *The Health Belief Model and Personal Health Behaviour*, Charles B. Slack, Thorofare, NJ.

Rudd, C., 2003, Merging general practice-driven reforms and public sector strategies in the 1990s: A framework for health policy, unpublished doctoral dissertation, University of Western Australia, Perth.

Shu, L.L., Gino, F., & Bazerman, M.H., 2009, *Dishonest Deed, Clear Conscience: Self-Preservation through Moral Disengagement and Motivated Forgetting (Working Paper)*, Harvard Business School, Boston, Massachusetts.

Singhal, A., Cody, M.J., Rogers, E., & Sabido, M., 2004, *Entertainment—Education and Social Change*, Lawrence Erlbaum Associates, Mahwah, NJ.

Spencer, L., Adams, T.B., Malone, S., Roy, L., & Yost, E., 2006, Applying the transtheoretical model to exercise: a systematic and comprehensive review of the literature, *Health Promot Pract* 7(4):428–43.

Squires, S., 2005, To lose well, think positive, *The Washington Post*, 22 March, p. HE01, www.washingtonpost.com/wp-dyn/articles/A55828-2005Mar22.html, accessed 23 March 2005.

Stokols, D., 1996, Translating social ecological theory into guidelines for community health promotion, *Am J Health Promot* 10(4):282–98.

Thaler, R., & Sunstein, C., 2008, *Nudge: Improving Decisions About Health, Wealth, and Happiness*, Yale University Press, New York.

Thomas, K., 1997, Health and morality in early modern England, in Brandt, A.M., & Rozin, P, (Eds.), *Morality and Health*, Routledge, New York, pp. 15–34.

Triandis, H.C., 1977, *Interpersonal Behaviour*, Brooks/Cole Publishing Company, Monterey, CA.

Tyler, T.R., 1990, *Why People Obey the Law*, Yale University Press, New Haven.

Tyler, T.R., 1997, Misconceptions about why people obey laws and accept judicial decisions, *American Psychological Society Observer* September, pp. 12–46.

Vila, B., 1994, A general paradigm for understanding criminal behaviour: extending evolutionary ecological theory, *Criminology* 32: 311–60.

Webb, T., & Sheeran, P., 2006, Does changing behavioural intentions engender behaviour change? A meta-analysis of the experimental evidence, *Psychol Bull* 132(2):249–68.

Whitelaw, S., MacHardy, L., Reid, W., & Duffy, M., 1999, The stages of change model and its use in health promotion: a critical review, Health Education Board of Scotland Research Centre.

WHO (World Health Organization), 2002, *World report on violence and health: Summary*, WHO, Geneva.

Yankelovich, D., 1992, How public opinion really works, *Fortune* 126(7):102–5.

chapter 3

Focus on the individual

Summary of main points

- Health promotion began as 'health education', in situations where the provision of information about health on a one-to-one basis was the focus (e.g. parent to child, midwife to expectant mother) and evolved over time into more formal clinical and educational applications.
- Individual approaches in clinical settings are usually, but not always, associated with secondary or tertiary prevention.
- Most individual approaches involve some form of one-to-one health counselling, for which outcomes can be improved by using special techniques, such as motivational interviewing.
- Primary health care, particularly in the context of a worldwide epidemic of chronic disease, is likely to play a much bigger role in health promotion.
- New technologies, including the internet, offer unique opportunities for access to individual information.
- Internet services such as 'Google Diagnosis' can be a two-edged sword: they can give individuals valuable information; however, they can be misused and the health information obtained can sometimes be unreliable.
- New opportunities exist for health promotion professionals to work at a clinical (one-to-one) level, dealing particularly with lifestyle and chronic diseases.

Why individual approaches?

An individual focus has been the cradle of health promotion. It is likely to have begun as the imparting of information about healthy living practices and the avoidance of health risks on a one-to-one basis: from mother to child, from midwife to mother and from doctor to patient. The influence of a credible personal source of health information remains strong and should not be undervalued, although a number of factors have changed the emphasis on this in recent times:

- With large populations, the intended audience is so numerous that it is too labour-intensive to reach everyone in this manner. In a traditional village, with extended families and a close interpersonal communication network, an individual focus might have been plausible. In a modern industrialised society, not only is it difficult to gain access to people but also health information is competing with a myriad of other messages, often from anti-health forces.
- Most information concerning health is now so technical and complex that a 'translation' process is necessary to transform scientific and medical terminology into information that can be understood and acted on by the general public.
- The advent of the internet has meant that easy access to wide-ranging health information is now available at the click of a mouse. This makes information transmission much quicker and easier (although the reliability of some health information accessed on the internet is of variable value).

Although an individual health promotion practitioner, even in a small community, would face a daunting task in counselling each individual in that community, there are many opportunities to reach individuals through other means: for example, enlisting various professionals who deal with people on a personal basis to incorporate health promotion into their role. In this way, the health promotion practitioner could facilitate the health promotion role of other health professionals. For example, an estimated 80 per cent of people visit a general practitioner (GP) as their first reference for health matters, and many regard their GP as their most influential source of information. There is therefore potential for involving the GP in health promotion. With the changing nature of disease, there has also been a rise in new health practitioners—such as lifestyle counsellors, life coaches, personal trainers, practice nurses and weight loss specialists—to help deal with contemporary health problems, particularly chronic diseases and their risk factors.

Individual methods in health promotion have limitations, particularly time and cost-effectiveness. However, the interactive nature of face-to-face communication allows greater possibilities for personal influence and potential lifestyle change than perhaps any other communication medium. There exists the notion of the 'teachable moment' (Lawson & Flocke 2009), which refers to the time or occasion when adopting positive changes in beliefs, attitudes and behaviours becomes possible or easiest. This can occur as a result of a crisis event or experience, such as a health scare, or death of a loved one from a particular health problem, which can then heighten the awareness of the individual to learning more about the situation and future prevention.

Individual methods

One of the most common individual methods in prevention is that which is generally referred to as 'patient education'. This reflects the fact that individual methods of health promotion are usually, but not exclusively, associated with either secondary prevention (i.e. attempts to reverse the early symptoms of disease) or tertiary prevention (i.e. attempts to slow the progress of a disease that already exists, such as after a heart attack).

On the other hand, individual risk factor assessment and identification can be regarded as secondary prevention (where illness risks are identified) or primary prevention (intervention aimed at avoiding illness before any disease state or symptoms exist). The common and important problem of hypertension (high blood pressure) offers a good example of primary, secondary and tertiary prevention:

- Primary prevention is education about avoiding obesity and inactivity, which can lead to hypertension.
- Secondary prevention is the detection and treatment of high blood pressure so as to avoid heart disease or stroke.
- Tertiary prevention is action, including medication, to prevent recurrence of a stroke or heart attack (in this case associated with hypertension). This can include rehabilitation after such events.

The escalation of chronic disease in the health burden has heightened the need for patient/health practitioner interactions, except that these days the practitioner may not be a doctor, but a practice nurse, allied health practitioner or a 'new' health professional such as a health coach or personal trainer. More commonly also, practitioners will work in teams, providing different expertise as required at different levels of intervention.

One-to-one individual methods are not as appropriate in the area of primary prevention, because of the cost incurred in reaching individuals in large populations, many of whom might never develop the specific disease. For this situation, group and whole-population approaches, aimed at making small health gains across larger populations, are more suitable. These will be discussed in Chapter 4.

Health literacy

A (previously understated) limiting factor in all forms of health management has been the health literacy of the client or patient. The most widely used definition of health literacy is: *'the degree to which individuals have the capacity to obtain, process and understand basic health information and services needed to make appropriate health decisions'* (Ratzan & Parker 2000). More operationally, it has been defined as *'a shared responsibility between patients (or anyone at the receiving end of health communication) and providers (or anyone on the giving end of health communication). Both must communicate in ways the other can understand'* (Osborne 2012). New findings that have come to light over the last decade or so suggest that up to 50 per cent of the population are 'health illiterate' (Nutbeam 2009) and this figure is even higher among the elderly, lower socioeconomic groups, and those from non-English speaking and Indigenous backgrounds.

Being aware of the potential problem of health literacy is important for health promotion personnel working at all levels. Full texts are now being published on the topic (e.g. Osborne 2012) and much research is being carried out both on ways of recognising health illiteracy, and helping overcome this through processes such as those defined through the acronym STEPS (Speak slowly, Teach back, Encourage questions, use Plain language and Show examples). In preparing health information, develop materials in different forms targeted at a health literacy around a late primary school level; these should be easily accessible for patients so they avoid the embarrassment of having to ask.

Patient education

Philosophy

Patient education can be classified according to who delivers the education (e.g. nurses, doctors, community health workers), the type of ailment involved (e.g. diabetes, heart disease, cancer), the intended audience (e.g. the elderly, mothers, mothers-to-be), where the education is delivered (e.g. hospital, medical or allied health professional settings) and the type of educational process (e.g. programmed learning, self-care, distance education). The primary philosophy is that patient education should:

- be integrated into patient care
- be developed in conjunction with patients
- include interdisciplinary involvement
- have specific and measurable goals.

In addition, patient education programs should involve families, partners and friends, as well as the patients themselves. The discussion below is categorised into settings in which patient education can occur. For more detailed information on patient education, readers are referred to the work of Redman (2001); Harris, Smith and Veale (2005); Falvo (2004); and Friedman and colleagues (2011).

Hospital settings

The historical role of hospital involvement in health promotion goes back to the beginnings of health care. As knowledge about the causes of disease increased, it became incumbent upon hospitals to try to reduce illness through programs aimed at the root causes of these illnesses. Initially, only first-aid classes were offered, but these have expanded to include many types of programs at both the inpatient and outpatient levels. Rapidly increasing health costs and the need for more beds has meant earlier discharge and hence the rise of outpatient programs such as Hospital in the Home (e.g. see health.vic.gov.au/hith). This has been enhanced by improvements in diagnostic and treatment technology, which have provided better information on which to base discharge.

Inpatient programs

Hospital inpatient programs are based on the premise that patients have a right to know not only the current status of their health but also what they can do to improve it and to prevent recurrences of illness. Inpatient programs can include:

- provision of appropriate health information
- a brief intervention by a health professional with an inpatient who presents with risk factors, or
- a specific intervention, such as a nurse-facilitated smoking cessation program in surgical pre-admission clinics (Haddock & Burrows 1997).

Inpatient programs can include general health education material (e.g. maintaining a healthy lifestyle) or education for specific ailments (e.g. diabetes, asthma, heart disease). These programs can include audiovisual resources, lecture, discussions, one-to-one counselling and printed materials, such as brochures and pamphlets. Depending on the client group, multilingual services might be required, in which case the health promotion practitioner could act as a coordinator of services rather than a deliverer. Media skills can be useful to develop audiovisual material, which might be specific to a particular inpatient situation or available for more general use. Multimedia resources are now also available commercially. Hospital libraries might hold many of these for loans.

Hospital staff support for health promotion activities with patients is generally high, particularly in the more commonly seen areas of smoking cessation and skin cancer prevention. However, sufficient funding, support from relevant personnel and availability of resources and training appear to be barriers to more hospital-based health promotion activities being undertaken.

The role of the health promotion practitioner in patient education includes the following:

- identifying the health problems that are amenable to education intervention
- formulating patient education goals and policies
- planning a course of action appropriate to these needs and goals
- determining the health behaviour and actions of patients that contributed to their specific health problems

- evaluating the education interventions to see whether they made a difference to a patient's health status
- planning staff development programs for health providers and other members of the health team on learning strategies and methods
- helping select, prepare and distribute educational materials to be used in patient education programs.

Resources of hospitals and clinics have historically been barely sufficient to allow them to carry out the curative and palliative care that the public demands. In this context, the diversion of resources or allocation of additional funding to the area of health promotion might sometimes be greeted less than enthusiastically by hospital and medical administrators. However, the opportunity to reach a 'captive' audience—with a vested interest in avoiding a recurrence of their illness—is one that offers challenges for the health promotion practitioner. Not the least of these is the problem of patient adherence to preventive practices once the patient has returned to their normal life (see Case study 3.1).

A relatively new process for hospital inpatient education is the use of a wide range of media that provide information about self-management and ongoing care. This ranges from simple video/TV programs to social media and applications for electronic tables. Triaging for certain conditions (i.e. chronic pain) also means that referrals can be made to less intensive treatments where this is indicated with a greater range of health promotion materials.

CASE STUDY 3.1

Nurse–patient effects on diabetes management

Lack of compliance with diabetes advice and prescription is a common problem, and complications often develop quickly. Researchers in the Netherlands tested adherence to a set of guidelines proposed for diabetes care in the hospital setting when these were imparted by doctors, nurses or other hospital staff. Compliance was greatest when a specialist diabetic nurse was used for patient education, which suggests that the selection of health promotion personnel could be just as important as the information imparted, if not more important. Specialist nurses obviously have the skills and time to ensure greater compliance with the message than other health personnel.

Dijkstra et al. 2004

Outpatient settings

Outpatient visits to hospitals outnumber inpatient experiences by a factor of approximately 10 to 1. Non-hospital care is likely to increase even further with current economic pressure on healthcare funding and the consequent move to alternative healthcare settings and arrangements, such as day surgeries, short-stay clinics and managed care organisations including health-maintenance organisations (HMOs). Therefore outpatient services represent a useful mode of health promotion intervention.

Outpatient services are frequently used by the elderly and the disadvantaged, as well as by many who don't necessarily use clinical care as much as social support services (e.g. alcohol and drug dependent persons, domestic violence cases) and who, by using these services, can overload their capacity and restrict availability to those more in need. Because clients from disadvantaged groups often frequent them, they can also be a setting for addressing social needs of individuals and possibly their neighbourhoods. For example, Roberts and colleagues (1995), in a study of 293 chronically ill patients attending outpatient clinics in Ontario, Canada, found that those who were poorly socially adjusted and who lived alone significantly improved their adjustment to illness and had fewer health service expenditures if they received problem-solving counselling.

A number of factors need to be taken into consideration in planning health promotion programs for outpatient facilities. These include:

- the characteristics of the outpatient staff (number, type, cooperation, time availability)
- the characteristics of the outpatient population (readiness to learn, number, type)
- the contact time of staff and patients
- availability of space
- availability and appropriateness of resources (e.g. audiovisual equipment).

Inpatient and outpatient programs should be complementary. Hence the latter might also involve:

- the use of multimedia resources
- the introduction of inpatient information needed to assist discharge and recovery
- printed or web-based materials with information on general and specific needs
- advice to and training of staff for basic outpatient counselling and delivery.

Because patient involvement could be high in relation to messages that relate directly and immediately to their own health outcomes, outpatient departments can make use of on-the-spot educational materials such as pamphlets, educational videos and user-friendly computer programs and interactive kiosks.

Group programs can also be run in both the inpatient and the outpatient setting. Group classes, support sessions, community seminars and health fairs are all methods that have been tried with varying degrees of success. Examples of health problems addressed by patient education programs include diabetes, asthma, heart disease, stroke, obesity and mental illness.

Lifestyle medicine

Lifestyle medicine is a new approach to dealing with lifestyle as a prominent cause of disease in modern times. Although it began in the US, with postgraduate medical training in three major universities (Harvard, Florida and Loma Linda) around the turn of the century, it has been progressed significantly through work in Australia. Lifestyle medicine is defined as '*the application of environmental, behavioural, medical and motivational principles (including self care and self-management) to the management of lifestyle-related health problems in a clinical setting*' (Egger, Binns & Rossner 2011). The availability of the chronic disease management system (CDMS) instituted by the Australian Government, involving a range of different health disciplines in a Medicare-funded process, has facilitated and embedded a lifestyle medicine approach to care within healthcare delivery. The inclusion of 'environmental principles' has also widened the scope of the discipline to be not just clinical, but to form a bridge between public health and clinical medicine. This recognises that the causes of modern disease are not just within the control of an individual's lifestyle choices, but more extant in the social, political and economic spheres.

Lifestyle medicine is predicated around the notion that ~70 per cent of modern diseases are of a chronic nature with a lifestyle and/or environmental aetiology (see Chapter 1). Its enactment involves not only the *content* of lifestyle and behavioural issues (i.e. knowledge about nutrition, physical activity, sleep, stress, drug and alcohol use, and social relations), but the *process* of how this is imparted through such techniques as health coaching, cognitive behaviour therapy, behaviour modification, motivational interviewing, group dynamics and self-management training.

Lifestyle medicine is not meant to replace the current medical model, but rather complement this with new techniques and information for dealing with more long-term care needs. Because of its nature, lifestyle medicine will increasingly require the input of health promotion professionals, not just at the 'front end' of health care (i.e. primary prevention), but in the secondary and tertiary requirements for self-care and self-management, which are set to become the mainstays of chronic disease management.

Self-care and self-management education

Because chronic disease, by definition, is long term, and because clinicians are unable to spend continual time with chronic disease sufferers, more needs to be done in the areas of self-care and self-management by the patients themselves. However, in a cyclical irony that defines modern health care, clinicians need to be taught how to teach their patients how do this.

The movement for self-care began in the 1970s. This initially referred to primary prevention—looking after oneself in order not to become ill.

Self-management became more prominent around the end of the millennium as a means of assisting patients to deal with existing chronic diseases. Initially this was not integrated into organised medical care programs. More recently, though, a systematised approach has been taken to reintegrate it into the health system and a number of structured approaches have been developed (e.g. see Egger, Binns & Rossner 2012, Chapter 5).

Diabetes self-management programs, for example, are now integrated into many clinical practices' guidelines and policies, and have become a prime focus for diabetes treatment. These involve educational programs designed to empower individuals to promote health and prevent adverse sequelae from their disease, as well as teach them how to interact effectively with the health system, monitor their physical and emotional status and make appropriate management decisions on the basis of the results of self-monitoring (Nuovo et al. 2007).

Self-management concentrates on three main tasks (medical, role and emotional management) and six main skills (problem solving, decision making, resource utilisation, the formation of a patient–provider partnership, action planning and self tailoring). The mechanism through which this has been evaluated as having a positive effect on health outcomes is by improving self-efficacy in the patient (Lorig & Holman 2003).

Counselling, brief interventions and motivational interviewing

Counselling is a form of systematic guidance offered by health professionals in which a person's problems are discussed and advice given. Most of the methods discussed here involve some form of counselling, and counselling can include a range of different principles and techniques. Brief interventions are a form of counselling aimed at making the most of any opportunity to raise awareness, share information and get a person thinking about making changes to his or her health-related behaviour. A clinician seeing a patient for an unrelated matter, for example, might note that the patient has gained significant weight or has taken up smoking since a previous visit, and then proceed to raise awareness about the related health risks and offer advice for dealing with them. The clinician or health professional delivering the brief intervention does not always have to be a doctor; in some cases, such as for some Aboriginal and Torres Strait Islander people, a health worker from their own culture may be better placed to deliver the health promotion message. For example, Hearn and colleagues (2011) showed that a training program designed for Aboriginal health workers and other health professionals working with Aboriginal clients to deliver a culturally specific, evidence-based brief smoking cessation intervention had an impact on the knowledge, skills and confidence of participants.

Telephone counselling has now become a significant means of assisting self-management, with several health insurance companies and their operatives using the process to reduce cost. Healthways, for example, is a US-based operation that has expanded to Australia to offer support for health insurance clients with long-term chronic disease. Trained counsellors provide ongoing support and assistance to individuals in the workplace, at home or in the process of moving from hospital to home care (see www.healthwaysaustralia. com.au). Other health insurance organisations in Australia are also adopting this approach to try to achieve a healthier client population and thereby reduce health costs (and health insurance claims), at least from chronic disease.

Motivational interviewing is a process of questioning that can be used effectively in counselling to raise a patient's likelihood of complying with a clinician's prescription. Motivational interviewing has a structured format that can be taught to clinicians and other health professionals (Miller & Rollnick 2002). This now forms a significant part of self-management education.

CASE STUDY **3.2**

Targeting behaviour change

Scottish exercise researcher Alison Kirk used motivational interviewing to target messages for diabetes patients identified as being in one of the first three levels of 'stages of change' (see Chapter 2) to become more physically active. A control group was given only standard advice on treatment for their disease. After 6 months the targeted group had not only considerably increased their level of physical activity as measured by movement sensors but had also increased their fitness, reduced their blood sugars (as measured by HbA1C) and improved their blood lipids. They had also shifted along the 'stages of change' in line with an improvement in motivation.

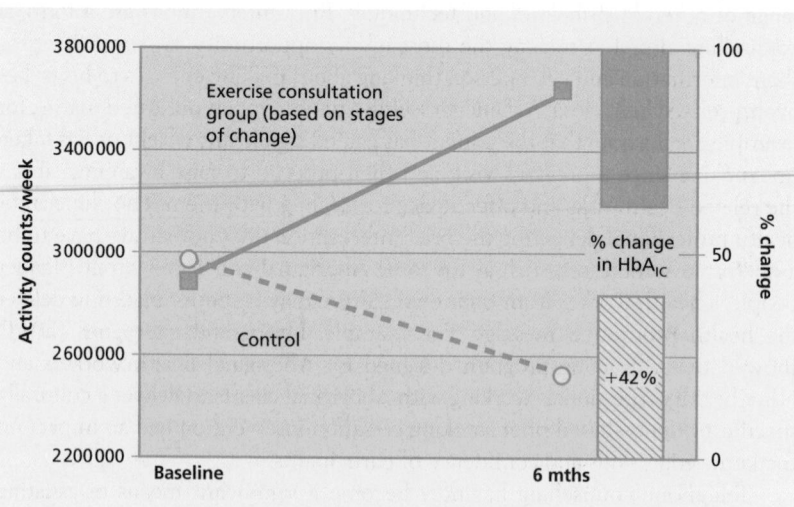

Figure 3.1: Increased activity and decreased HbA1C in diabetics given exercise prescription based on stages of change

From Kirk et al. 2003

Primary health care

'Primary health care' refers to policies formalised in the Declaration of Alma Ata in 1978, and subsequently adopted by the World Health Organization (WHO) and other United Nations organisations.

Primary health care is concerned with the first level of the health system: the initial point of contact for people seeking assistance with a health problem or for general health-related advice. As this level of service requires structures to integrate with each other and the whole health system, primary health care is also an approach to service delivery.

The primary healthcare approach comprises a set of principles, including:

- intersectoral collaboration
- coordination of primary, secondary and tertiary health services to facilitate continuity of care
- balanced resource use addressing both intermediate needs and longer term issues
- a population focus, with special attention to high-risk and vulnerable groups as a precondition for equity in health outcomes and healthcare access
- appropriate technology (WHO 1983).

As a signatory to this global policy direction, Australia has seen this commitment articulated in state and national health policies. These policy initiatives have led to the growth of primary healthcare centres and the establishment of university-based centres of excellence in primary health care.

Health promotion is a key strategy of primary healthcare practitioners, particularly through:

- health promotion planning that facilitates community involvement in the identification of priorities and the ownership of programs
- the provision of intersectoral advocacy for healthy public policy
- the delivery of interactive health education.

Although it is important that primary health care is adopted within secondary and tertiary healthcare settings, the community health services sector provides the leading edge for implementation of primary health care, owing mainly to its collaboration in defined localities or neighbourhoods. Other groups to be considered under this heading are doctors, practice nurses and other allied health professionals.

Community health centres

Within any community, community health services combine health promotion, early detection and intervention, rehabilitation and the management of chronic health problems. Established in Australia in the 1970s, community health centres—providing accessible, primary health care in a user-friendly, multipurpose setting—are logical venues for all levels of preventive intervention in individual and group settings. The health centre can also be a venue for community development action, which stimulates programs from the ground up.

Community health centres are often the source of much health information material and/or have access to central library facilities. Individual counselling, risk factor assessment and audiovisual education can be carried out in the health centre setting, including programs covering:

- relationship counselling, maternal and child health, crisis counselling
- psychological assessments and early interventions
- chronic disease care
- care coordination and counselling.

CASE STUDY **3.3**

Focusing on mothers

Historically, prenatal care and health promotion has been concerned with delivering a good birth outcome (such as ideal birthweight) for the infant.

This was (rightly) aimed at reducing the high rates of infant mortality associated with early and pre-developed societies. However, while infant mortality rates have improved dramatically, at least in non-Indigenous populations, there has been a shift of focus away from the health of the mother, resulting in big increases in gestational diabetes mellitus (GDM), which can progress to later type 2 diabetes. In Pacific Island cultures in particular, adoption of European approaches to childbirth has meant a significant decrease in activity levels of new mothers and an excessive fat gain as they are 'wrapped in cotton-wool' by relatives to ensure a good birth outcome.

Recent attention has therefore been given to exercise and diet programs in pregnancy, with the goal of remaining active and not gaining excessive weight. Because of the value of exercise in maintaining blood sugar levels, innovative programs using aerobics, aquarobics and resistance training are now being promoted. Research on resistance training using rubber bands has shown a decrease in the effects of GDM from 26 to 32 weeks of pregnancy compared with a standard recommended diet program. This, and other recent work showing the reversibility of early stage type 2 diabetes with lifestyle change, is likely to change the nature of antenatal health promotion in the future. Marriage and pregnancy in island and Indigenous cultures offer ideal opportunities for focusing pre- and postnatal health promotion messages aimed at ensuring the health of the mother, as well as the baby.

Medical and allied professional programs

These programs consist of patient education services provided by doctors, dentists, physiotherapists, dietitians, podiatrists, occupational therapists and other health professionals. Because time is often limited, the most effective vehicle for health promotion is a brief, or 'low intensity' intervention supported by relevant resources and information.

General medical practice

General medical practice is the first point of contact with the healthcare system for the majority of people in Australia. More than 85 per cent of the population visit a GP at least once a year and, on average, people visit a GP approximately five times each year (AIHW 2012). It is estimated that up to 60 per cent of attendances at general practice are precipitated by a lifestyle-based—and hence predominantly preventable—cause (AIHW 2012). However, a range of professional, regulatory and health sector financing issues, along with various political and social trends, have been impediments to general practice realising its full potential in the Australian healthcare system (ACHR 2011).

The General Practice Strategy, introduced by the Australian Government in 1992 and since updated, aimed to improve access to general practice services, encourage the improved integration of general practice with the rest of the healthcare system, enhance the quality and cost-effectiveness of general practice, and support training for GPs (DHSH 1996). The strategy included the establishment of networks of GPs, to reduce the sense of professional isolation experienced by GPs, who are often excluded from involvement in hospital care, teaching, research and local or regional health planning. These networks—known as divisions of general practice—provided infrastructure and funding that enabled GPs to undertake cooperative activities to improve their integration with other elements of the health system.

More recently (from 1 July 2011), around 160 divisions of general practice around Australia were combined into 61 larger areas called Medicare Locals. These were established to coordinate primary healthcare delivery and tackle local healthcare needs and service gaps by providing a broader range of providers and activities. Medicare Locals are intended to drive improvements in primary health care and ensure that services are better tailored to meet the needs of local communities. Key roles identified for such networks/organisations are 'health promotion, illness prevention and population health activities at the local level, including coordination of general practitioners' participation in regional and national programs' (Medicare Locals 2011).

In line with international trends to address equity in health outcomes in developed nations, funding has been provided to make general practice health promotion and other activities a reality. This finance will encourage population-based planning, which identifies long-term goals and specific target areas in which maximum health gains can be achieved. The improved integration of GPs into healthcare teams that include health professionals with specific skills in different areas has increased the possibility of greater health promotion in clinical practice. Practice nurses, who are currently the fastest growing profession in the country, are now more available to assist GPs in much of the detailed educational and support work that GPs have little time to do.

General practice continues to provide an important and cost-effective setting for health promotion because of the high patient-contact rates and the credibility of GPs as perceived by the public. For example, smoking intervention programs administered by GPs have resulted in significant reductions in smoking (Richards et al. 2003). The majority of patients considered that their chances of success were greater if a doctor administered the smoking intervention programs, and that having the results of lung function and blood tests (explained in relation to the risks of cardiovascular and respiratory diseases) constituted a strong incentive to stop smoking. GP patient education has also demonstrated success with many other health problems over the years, including HIV/AIDS (Gallagher 1989), back pain (Roland & Dixon 1989), hypertension (Watkins et al. 1987) and the reduction of excessive alcohol consumption (Wallace, Cutler & Haines 1988; Richmond et al. 1998).

In relation to patient information, the new and bigger general practices and super-clinics arising around the country are more able to act as a 'hub' within a 'hub and spoke' type approach to providing health information. Much generalised information, including brochures, posters and information sheets, can come from the practice 'hub', whereas 'spokes' can include more specialised services such as self-help groups, internet sites, community health centres, libraries, video services and other allied care referrals.

Because clinical health professionals may have limited knowledge and training in health promotion, the possibility of health promotion specialist support to such clinicians could be yet another method of getting information to the public. Exercise, stress management and alcohol and drug education are areas in which clinical health professionals accept their educational limitations and, in some cases, welcome complementary expertise. Health promotion practitioners could consider using the increasing interest shown by Medicare Locals in developing continuing professional development (CPD) training for GPs and allied health professionals in a range of issues, but particularly relating to chronic disease management.

Allied health professionals

A number of contemporary disciplines now exist to aid health promotion at the clinical level. In addition to traditional disciplines such as dietitians, psychologists, podiatrists and physiotherapists, newer professional roles include practice nurses within medical surgeries, lifestyle counsellors, life coaches, health coaches and personal trainers. Under the government policy for utilising allied health professionals, which has resulted in the development of Medicare Locals and a rise in GP super-clinics, personnel trained in these areas work in an integrated clinical team alongside GPs to provide lifestyle programs to patients with metabolic and lifestyle-related disorders, such as obesity, diabetes and heart disease. This offers new career opportunities in health promotion for those who might choose to work at the clinical (one-to-one) level rather than at the population level.

Pharmacies

The potential of pharmacies as health promotion outlets is only beginning to be realised. In some states, health insurance companies are utilising pharmacies as an outlet for summary information sheets, which also advertise the company's services. As shelf space is a priority in pharmacies, special pamphlet racks are provided by the companies.

Pharmacy Self-Care Fact Cards and self-help, touch-service computer programs were developed by the Pharmaceutical Society of Australia as part of its Pharmacy Self-Care Program.

Pharmacies are also becoming involved in risk factor screening for such problems as osteoporosis (Goode, Swiger & Bluml 2004) and smoking cessation (Sinclair, Bond & Stead 2004) as well as other forms of health promotion (Chandra, Malcolm & Fetters 2003. They are being used as a primary care service system (Carmichael et al. 2004), even including providing immunisations in some areas.

Home healthcare providers

With growing concern about hospital costs and an increasingly ageing population, there is increasing demand for home-based health care. Research with aged people has shown that better health outcomes are achieved when people can remain in their homes and get outside help. Usually these services come from the ranks of nursing and are employed by government, local hospitals or community and non-governmental organisations (e.g. Blue Care, Silver Chain). However, there is an increasing trend towards privately run home-care services.

The opportunity for home-care patient education is likely to increase as the ageing population becomes more e-literate and able to access health programs on the internet. This is likely to be aimed mainly at seniors and, to a lesser extent, people with a disability. Areas for development include nutrition, exercise, prevention of trauma and other aspects of self-care, such as preventing falls. Intervention could consist of written and electronic material, but is more likely to include some form of one-to-one counselling. The health promotion practitioner in these settings could act as a trainer of the home-care provider in health promotion skills.

The increasing use of information and communications technology in health has also signalled a potential expansion of home care with home monitoring of vital signs for patients with chronic disease. Home visits by nurses in person can be replaced by telemedicine videophone consultations (Celler, Lovell & Basilakis 2003). Pharmacies are also becoming more involved in 'outreach' services where they go to patients, rather than vice versa.

Self-help materials and the internet

'Programmed learning' refers to learning carried out in a sequential pattern. It is generally computer-based or by means of written, structured manuals, and is often used for individualised education and change, particularly for patient education and professional training programs.

Internet

The introduction of computers has led to computer-aided instruction, and the internet is available at the click of a mouse. Patients are able to get readily available, free information about areas of particular interest just by using search engines, thus placing additional pressure on medical practitioners, for whom one topic is only a small area of their knowledge base. Easier access to information is changing the nature of medical practice and necessitating greater specialty areas, such as the allied health professionals referred to above. Despite the huge variation in the relevance and quality of internet-based health information and programs, it is clear that e-health is now a major part of the answer to treating chronic disease in Australia and a key factor in reducing the considerable costs (ACHR 2011).

CASE STUDY **3.4**

Self-help websites: the depression example

Although website health information is often variable, it is difficult to find a reliable, user-friendly but evidence-based site. The Black Dog Institute (www.blackdoginstitute. org.au) and *beyondblue* (www.beyondblue.org.au) provide excellent information for people with depression anxiety or a related disorder, their family and friends.

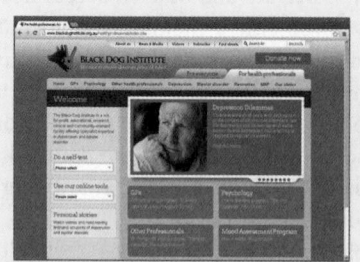 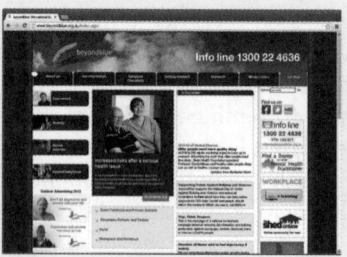

Courtesy of the Black Dog Institute and beyondblue

Despite the wide proliferation of services, there is little evidence of the effects of the internet on healthcare outcomes (Bessell et al. 2002). The challenge is to equip consumers with the knowledge and discriminatory skill to appraise information selectively.

New technology has also led to the development of social media with potential for health promotion that has yet to be realised (Grossberndt, van den Hazel & Bartonova 2012). Facebook, SMS and Twitter all offer opportunities for individual health communication and social marketing, as discussed in Chapter 5. Webinars, e-newsletters and a range of new techniques are also available or on the horizon, and may offer opportunities as well as challenges in the future because of the diverse range of communication options available.

Email

Email, which is now one of the more established communication forms despite the relatively short time interval since the introduction of the internet in the mid-1990s, has opened up opportunities for delivering information to large numbers of individuals at the click of a mouse. Previously this required the printing, layout, publishing and postage of materials, all of which are costly and time-consuming. Email, however, allows distribution to be done simply and cheaply. Hence groups defined by certain interest areas can receive regular newsletters, updates, journal articles or other forms of support from an authoritative source. Email is also suggested as a possible future way for medical practice to involve patients in their own care and optimise face-to-face visits (Meyer 2004).

Programmed learning and distance learning health programs

Programmed learning works best when health promotion practitioners have the resources to produce their own educational modules and materials for a specific market. Consumer preferences indicate that programmed learning in the form of distance learning programs may be more desirable than face-to-face formats for some people, particularly more highly educated and higher-income groups (Sherwood et al. 1998). Programs can range from being totally self-help with minimal contact to adding a component to a shared care program. They have also been offered at no cost, at commercial rates or with different forms of cost incentive. Reported success rates are generally higher with some level of payment, perhaps indicating a level of self-selection through commitment.

Programmed instruction requires frequent use of materials and situations that are more appropriate for an individual approach rather than a group situation (e.g. in cases of geographic isolation or sensitivity). The use of programmed learning for smoking cessation and exercise instruction, for example, has been developed and evaluated in South Australia by Owen (1988).

Programmed learning is most appropriate when:

- the range of individual differences is great enough to require individual learning
- the topic is sensitive and calls for a degree of privacy (e.g. STIs)
- the subject material is straightforward and does not require clarification
- there are sufficient funds and support to ensure continuity of such a program.

Australia offers particular challenges for health promotion in the area of programmed learning because of the existence of rural and isolated people with specific health needs.

Health promotion shopfronts

Shopfront services for health promotion materials and programs have been tried in various cities (in the city centre or in major shopping malls) around the country. Although these are community based, the strategy is focused on large numbers of one-to-one interactions.

The first test of health promotion shopfronts was as part of the experimental North Coast Healthy Lifestyle program in 1978–81 in Lismore, New South Wales (Egger et al. 1983). Since then, shopfronts of various forms have been created throughout Australia, including those for non-government organisations, such as the Heart Foundation, cancer councils and Diabetes Australia.

Shopfronts are able to provide many of the services available in all forms of health promotion: literature, risk factor assessment, counselling, lectures, group programs, and computerised instruction and testing. Their major advantage is that they 'get in people's way', often while they are shopping, and so they can reach such groups as blue-collar workers or parents who might not seek health information and programs in formal healthcare settings or government offices. Shopfronts could also be a source of funds for an organisation, although commercial lease costs in central public access points, such as city malls and shopping centres, could be prohibitive.

The shopfront can be used as a source of two-way interaction in the health promotion process with clients contributing experiences and needs to staff, and programs being developed to cater for those needs. A shopfront can serve as a community focus for large-scale health promotion programs and campaigns and become a staging point for promotions, as well as a reference point for materials and information.

Because of the issues of cost and sustainability, health promotion shopfronts—pioneered by state and territory health departments in the 1970s and 1980s—are today more likely to be found within the operations of private sector health insurance organisations and/or pharmacies.

Risk factor assessments

As noted in the introduction to this chapter, risk factor assessment is usually used as a means of secondary prevention. However, in some cases (e.g. nutrition analysis, fitness assessment, body weight analysis, mental health strengths) it can be used in primary prevention to develop programs that could enable an individual to stay healthy. A number of risk factor assessments is currently available, and the form and source of some of these are listed below. Risk factor measurements can be carried out directly by an experienced health promotion practitioner; alternatively, the practitioner could facilitate assessments by other qualified health professionals.

Health risk appraisal

Health risk appraisals (HRAs) are available through a number of computerised tests that are often accessible via shopfront services or existing health-related outlets, such as pharmacies.

HRAs have limited validity because of the subjective nature of many of the questions. However, a study of the accuracy of HRAs in predicting mortality has shown that they could be appropriate for identifying high-risk populations for health interventions (Pai et al. 2009). They could also serve as a motivational starting point for some individuals by creating a perceived need for behaviour change.

Blood chemistry screening

Recent developments in blood chemistry have broadened the range of measures available for assessing risk (see box 'Risk measurements for the overweight'). Although most of these tests require sending blood to a pathology laboratory for testing, the development of dry chemistry processes for assessing blood lipids, and portable home devices for measuring blood sugars, now allow rapid and reasonably accurate measurements of cholesterol and some other plasma lipids.

Risk measurements for the overweight

Screening for health risk is useful for the overweight as being overweight is itself a health risk. Some simple measures that might be taken, their cut-off points and what they mean are shown below.

Waist circumference
Because abdominal fat is more dangerous than fat stored elsewhere, waist circumference is a good measure of health risk.

continued

continued

Desirable levels: less than 100 cm for Caucasian men and less than 90 cm for Caucasian women. The desirable level for Asians, Indians and Indigenous Australians is approximately 10 cm less and for Pacific Islanders approximately 10 cm more than these levels.

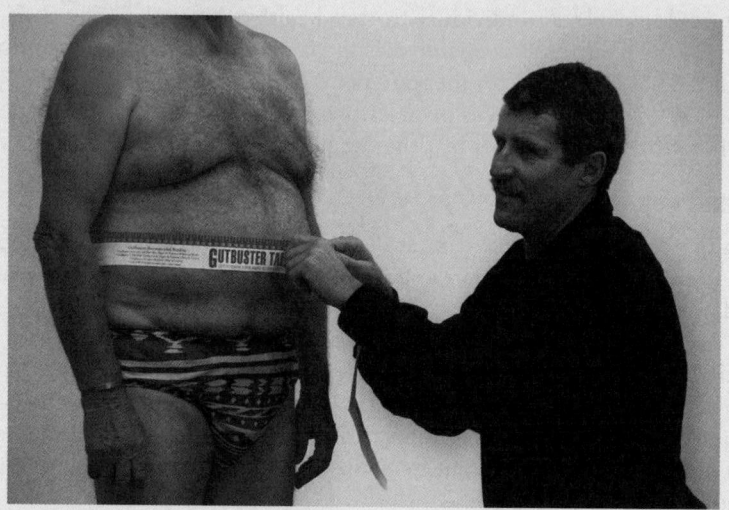

Measuring waist circumference   *Fairfax*

Body fat

Commercially available body weight scales are now able to per cent measure body fat in an individual. Bio-impedance analysis (BIA) measures are based on resistance to a small electric current that is passed around the body through the feet.

Desirable levels: recommended body fat levels for males are between 12 and 24 per cent of total body mass. Recommended levels for females are between 15 and 35 per cent.

Ideal body weight

A formula for measuring ideal body weight based on current weight and body fat percentage (as determined above) is:

$$\text{ideal weight} = \text{lean body weight} \div 1 - \text{desired fat \%}$$

This allows for gradual changes in goals based on moving towards a recommended body fat percentage.

Blood pressure

Blood pressure is likely to be increased with increased body fat. There is also a genetic component in cases of very high blood pressure, which requires medication. Mild increased blood pressure (hypertension) can be reduced with weight loss and, in particular, increased physical activity.

Desirable levels: less than 120/80 mmol/L

Cholesterol

Cholesterol is a waxy fat-like substance that can clog arteries. There are genetic influences, and total cholesterol is now considered to be only part of the story.
Desirable levels: less than 5.5 mmol/L. Sub-fractions include:
* LDL or 'bad' cholesterol—*Desirable levels:* less than 3.0 mmol/L
* HDL or 'good' cholesterol—*Desirable levels:* greater than 1.0 mmol/L

Triglyceride (Tg)

Tg is a combination of fats that are potentially dangerous, particularly in combination with a high waist circumference and high blood pressure and low HDL.
Desirable levels: less than 3.0 mmol/L

The 'triglyceride-waist' is a combination of these two measures: where waist circumference is above the recommended level and Tg is above 3 mmol/L. This is indicative of a fatty liver.

Fasting plasma glucose (FPG)

FPG is a measure of blood sugars indicating risk of diabetes.
Desirable levels: less than 5.5 mmol/L

HbA1C

HbA1C is a longer term measure of blood sugars over 3 to 6 months; less variable than FPG.
Desirable levels: less than 6 per cent

C-reactive protein (CRP)

CRP is a relatively new test, which measures inflammation and possible artery damage. These could be markers for heart disease and other health problems.

Mass cholesterol screening programs have been carried out in Australia and overseas. A large-scale screening demonstration program on the north coast of New South Wales was shown to be effective in identifying about a third of the population at risk of heart disease because of high cholesterol (James et al. 1989). The implications of the prevalence of high cholesterol for health promotion have been expounded by McMahon (1990), who suggested from a meta-analysis of epidemiological cholesterol studies that a 10 per cent reduction in cholesterol levels in the Australian population could result in the prevention of 20 000 deaths owing to heart disease per year.

Dietary assessment

By tradition, dietary assessment has been carried out by qualified dietitians in a clinical setting. The advent of computers and more precise nutrient details has meant the development of more reliable computerised nutrition assessment programs.

It is important to remember that nutrition assessments are diagnostic and require interpretation by a qualified professional. Although non-nutritionists could make assessments, any complete program should involve detailed counselling by an appropriate professional. Other means of testing dietary intake are: (a) the diet diary, (b) food recall, and (c) a food intake checklist. The latter can include a check of specific foods eaten such as dietary fat, carbohydrate or drinks, where these are perceived to be a potential problem.

Computerised diet checks—what comes out might not accurately reflect what goes in

Computers have been used in nutrition since the late 1950s, but the advent of personal computers in the 1980s has put computerised diet checks within reach of the ordinary home. A variety of nutrition analysis programs is now commercially available. The difficulty for someone not versed in nutrition and computers is how to choose. With prices ranging from a few dollars to several thousand, the wrong choice—for professional or personal use—can be costly.

Simplifying computers and diets

In simple terms, computers are a way of counting numbers or estimating quantities. Food is made up of various quantities of chemicals called nutrients. Some of these (e.g. carbohydrate, protein, fats) form a large or important component of most foods, and some (e.g. selenium, manganese) are important in particular foods.

Computers count the nutrients in the total diet by using information stored in a program database for a wide range of commonly eaten foods, and by multiplying the result by the foods eaten over a prespecified time period.

Although this is logically sound, there are a number of factors that can make or break a computer diet check. For example:

- *The information from which the database is derived might be spurious.* There are many sources of nutrient analysis, some more reliable than others. This should not be unexpected because the nutrient quantity of food can vary enormously depending on where it is grown, fertilisers used, climate and treatment (the vitamin A content of carrots, for example, can vary by 2500%, depending on variety and maturity). Standard nutrient analyses come from recognised government bodies such as the CSIRO or the US Department of Agriculture.
- *The database might not be big enough.* It is difficult to get accurate nutrient analyses for all the thousands of foods that people eat. The size of the database varies from 50 to 15 000 foods (obviously the bigger the database, the bigger the computer needed to store it). Usually between 1500 and 1800 items seems to be sufficient and manageable for most purposes.
- *The number of nutrients might be inadequate.* Some databases contain up to 50 nutrients, some of which are of little importance for most purposes.

The difficulty is that analyses on many of these nutrients (i.e. certain amino acids) do not exist for many of the foods in the database. Hence, total nutrient analysis can be misleading. The main requirements for general use are the macronutrients (carbohydrates, protein, fat), energy levels (calories or kilojoules), 8 to 10 vitamins (including A, B1, B2, B3, B6, B12, C, E, pantothenic acid) and 3 to 5 minerals (including Ca, An, Fe, Mg).

- *Input might be too complicated.* Input into most programs can be either in numbered codes (representing each food) or as food names. The more modern programs simply require typing the name of the food into the computer, and it is then recognised by the database. Where a food has several subcategories (e.g. corn: fresh cob, tinned, cream), the computer poses alternatives and a simple numbered response is required. Some programs have 'help' screens so that operations are user friendly.
- *Output might be inadequate.* Depending on the needs of the user, the output of a diet check program should be informative and educational. At least a printed output of major nutrients and a comparison with recommended daily requirements is required. This should be accompanied by a discussion about each of the critical nutrients in the diet and how the diet could be altered for improvement.
- *Individual differences might not be considered.* The metabolism of foods can vary between individuals and, although it is impossible to predict absorption rates for all nutrients, overall energy usage rates should be able to be measured and taken into consideration in the assessment of energy intake. At present, few diet check programs measure energy output, but those that do are becoming more common.

Fitness and activity assessments

Measuring fitness and activity levels can involve two separate components of measurement. Physical activity is usually measured using a recall or activity check questionnaire. More recently, the advent of pedometers and other movement sensors, which count the number of steps taken over the course of a day, have been used to measure baseline levels of activity as well as prescribe required amounts of activity for health and weight loss benefits.

Fitness assessments usually encompass more intrusive measures of physiological capacity. They can consist of a variety of subcomponents, including aerobic fitness, strength, body composition, flexibility, anthropometry and lung capacity. In general, these involve practical measurement techniques that should be performed by qualified exercise personnel (Egger, Champion & Bolton 1998). However, basic fitness testing can be carried out in many cases by trained sub-professional 'fitness leaders' and personal trainers, who might or might not be qualified health promotion practitioners.

Computerised scoring of fitness tests is also available, and it can vary from relatively cheap and simple programs to expensive, detailed, advanced versions.

Currently, computerised government fitness testing programs are not widely available, but departments of sport and recreation in most states are able to provide resources and information.

Fitness assessments can be carried out in commercial fitness centres, medical practices, community health centres, the workplace and even the home. Testing is usually used as a basis for developing individualised fitness programs, which again requires the skill of a qualified exercise professional. In some states, testing is now carried out by health insurance organisations and there are now several corporate health organisations that conduct fitness and other health testing in the workplace.

Testing 'signature strengths' and mental health

As part of the movement to positive psychology (Donovan & Egger 2011), Martin Seligman, one the founders of the movement in the US, has developed a test of 'signature strengths (see www.authentichappiness.com), which offers a short cut to identifying an individual's five most prominent strengths. These can then be focused on to improve satisfaction and quality of life and avoid depression. A full explanation of this is contained in the *Handbook of Signature Strengths* (Pearson & Seligman 2004).

In a similar vein, an online self-assessment tool for mental health activities is available within the Act Belong Commit mental health program (www.actbelongcommit.org.au) developed by Donovan and colleagues (2003).

Individual educational materials

Educational materials for patients and individuals can be in several forms. They can be informational (e.g. pamphlets—printed or electronic—on health and nutrition), prescriptional (e.g. nutrition for diabetics, exercise for cardiac rehabilitation), contractual (e.g. statement of intent to quit smoking) or evaluational (e.g. progress charts for weight control and stress management).

Much information is already available from various sources. Assessment of health educational material should be based on the following questions:

* *Does it appeal to the senses?* Good-quality educational material should be consonant with the aspirations and needs of the reader. It should look attractive and presentable and be easy to understand.
* *Is it culturally specific?* Material promoting the eating of pork is unlikely to be accepted in a large Jewish community, and the promotion of non-indigenous values might have little motivational value to Indigenous groups. Where possible, material should be produced within a culture itself and in the language of that culture. Kreuter and McClure (2004) suggest that culture is particularly relevant when considering the source, message and channel factors in communications.

- *Is the reading comprehension level appropriate?* It is a common axiom adopted by the popular press that the reading age of the average reader is around the early teens. Although this is not always so, it is true that it is a mistake to make over-optimistic assumptions about comprehension levels, even in professional groups. Of course, the reverse—that is, being patronising—is also a danger. This relates back to the importance of recognising the level of 'health literacy' as discussed earlier in this chapter.
- *Is the information accurate?* Health professionals and scientists are often pedantic about small matters that they have been involved with for many years. Materials should always be checked for accuracy with specialists in the field to avoid embarrassment once materials are released.
- *Does it achieve its objective?* The objective of any patient educational material needs to be clearly stated. Is it to provide knowledge, change attitudes or influence behaviour? Different objectives will influence both the presentation and the content of materials.

Existing educational resources

A range of patient education materials is available from government departments of health and community services. A variety of other materials can be readily and cheaply obtained online or in print form from a variety of sources, including:

- *Australian Lifestyle Medicine Association* (ALMA)—has downloadable fact sheets and patient tests available online (www.lifestylemedicine.com.au).
- *Heart Foundation* (Australia and New Zealand)—has materials on nutrition, heart disease and exercise.
- *State cancer councils*—have materials on all forms of cancer, smoking and nutrition.
- *State government departments of sport and recreation*—have materials on exercise, recreation and water safety.
- *Australian Nutrition Foundation*—has reliable information on nutrition
- *Private sector*—materials related to products being sold are available. Some might not be seen as impartial (e.g. information on sugar from the sugar industry), but others are prepared in conjunction with impartial bodies, such as the Royal Australian College of General Practitioners.
- *Health insurance organisations*—because they have a vested interest in keeping people well, these organisations are motivated to produce high-quality, useful health information.
- *Medical and pharmaceutical societies*—various medical and pharmaceutical societies and specialty groups (e.g. diabetes, asthma) produce accurate and useful information in the area; medical organisations have become increasingly active in producing health educational material, including videos.

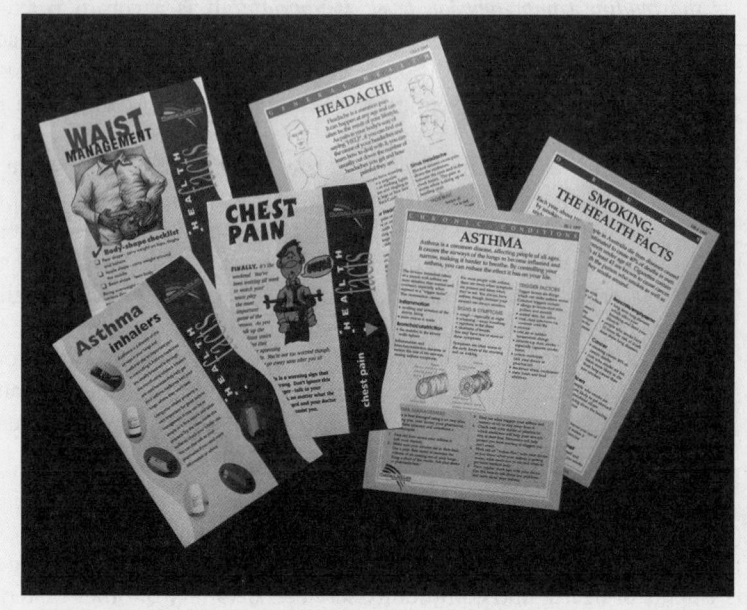

Fact cards from the Pharmacy Self-care Program

- *Professional associations*—professional organisations such as the Public Health Association of Australia and New Zealand and the Australian Council for Health, Physical Education and Recreation sometimes receive grants to produce materials in their area of expertise.
- *Private organisations*—there are health newsletters such as Health Yourself for industry and the Health Reader (produced by Choice) for the professional and interested lay reader; many health videos are now also available on loan from major video-hire outlets and libraries, and online.
- *Internet*—the health resources on the internet are multiplying at an extraordinary rate, although caution needs to be exercised in terms of depending on the source as this may not be valid.

Conclusion

Although the economics of health dictate that health promotion practitioners appeal to as wide an audience as possible, certain aspects of health promotion call for an individual focus. Patient education, although individual in orientation, also involves the development of materials with scope for wider usage. Other techniques, such as risk factor screening— although costly and time-consuming—are potentially useful tools for the health promotion practitioner, whether working in the individual, group or population-level setting.

Career opportunities in health promotion

The range of individual approaches considered here presents a variety of new and existing career options for health promotion practitioners. Clinical counselling is available through allied health professionals such as dietitians, psychologists, health coaches and evidence-based complementary medicine practitioners. However, there is a growing need for lifestyle and metabolic counsellors with knowledge in exercise, nutrition and psychology and skills in counselling to work in medical clinics and in shared care with other disciplines. Patient education is available in a number of different areas, including hospitals, community health centres, home care and private consulting. Patient education can also include health professional—or 'train-the-trainer'—options, such as teaching of doctors, nurses, fitness leaders and other health specialists about lifestyle-based health. New opportunities exist in developing internet sites and programmed learning for specialist areas, such as diabetes, weight control and heart disease, and this could be done with the aid of sponsors or on a fee-for-service basis. Risk factor analysis and health programming are further specialties developed in particular by personal trainers and lifestyle counsellors.

References

ACHR (Australian Centre for Health Research), 2011, *Health Care in Australia: Prescriptions for Improvement*, ACHR, Melbourne.

AIHW (Australian Institute of Health and Welfare), 2004, *The Burden of Disease and Injury in Australia*, AIHW, Canberra.

AIHW (Australian Institute of Health and Welfare), 2012, *Australia's Health 2012*, Australia's health series no. 13, Cat. no. AUS 156, AIHW, Canberra.

Bessell, T.L., McDonald, S., Silagy, C.A., Anderson, J.N., Hiller, J.E., & Sansom L.N., 2002, Do internet interventions for consumers cause more harm than good? A systematic review, *Health Expect* 2002;5(1):28–37.

Carmichael, J.M., Alvarez, A., Chaput, R., DiMaggio, J., Magallon, H., & Mambourg, S., 2004, Establishment and outcomes of a model primary care pharmacy service system, *Am J Health Syst Pharm* 61(5):472–82.

Celler, B.G., Lovell, N.H., & Basilakis, J., 2003, Using information technology to improve the management of chronic disease, *Med J Aust* 179:242–5.

Chandra, A., Malcolm, N., & Fetters, M., 2003, Practicing health promotion through pharmacy counseling activities, *Health Prom Pract* 4(1):64–71.

DHSH (Department of Human Services and Health), 1996, *Fact Sheets on General Practice*, DHSH, Canberra.

Dijkstra, R.F., Braspenning, J.C., Huijsmans, Z., Peters, S., van Ballegooie, E., ten Have, P., Casparie, A.F., & Grol, R.P., 2004, Patients and nurses determine variation in adherence to guidelines at Dutch hospitals more than internists or settings, *Diabet Med* 21(6):586–91.

Donovan, R.J., & Egger, G., 2011, Mental healthiness: the flip side of S-AD, in Egger, G., Binns, A. & Rossner, S. (Eds) *Lifestyle Medicine*, McGraw-Hill, Sydney.

Donovan, R.J., Watson, N., Henley, N., Williams, A., Silburn, S., Zubrick, S., James, R., Cross, D., Hamilton, G., & Roberts, C., 2003, *Mental Health Promotion Scoping Project. Report to Healthway*, Centre for Behavioural Research in Cancer Control, Curtin University, Western Australia.

Egger, G., Binns, A., & Rossner, S., 2012, *Lifestyle Medicine: Managing Diseases of Lifestyle in the 21st Century* (2nd edn), McGraw-Hill, Sydney.

Egger, G., Champion, C.N., & Bolton, A., 1998, *The Fitness Leader's Handbook* (3rd edn), Kangaroo Press, Sydney.

Egger, G., Fitzgerald, W., Frape, G., Monaem, A., Rubinstein, P., Tyler, C., & Mackay, B., 1983, Results of a large-scale media anti-smoking campaign in Australia: the North Coast Healthy Lifestyle Programme, *BMJ* 287:1125–87.

Falvo, D.R., 2004, *Effective Patient Education: A Guide to Increased Compliance* (3rd edn), Jones & Bartlett, Sudbury, Massachusetts.

Friedman, A.J., Cosby, R., Boyko, S., Hatton-Bauer, J., & Turnbull, G., 2011, Effective teaching strategies and methods of delivery for patient education: a systematic review and practice guideline recommendations, *J Cancer Educ* 26(1):12–21.

Gallagher, M., 1989, HIV prevention in general practice, *Practitioner* 233:942–3.

Goode, J.V., Swiger, K., & Bluml, B.M., 2004, Regional osteoporosis screening, referral, and monitoring program in community pharmacies: findings from Project ImPACT: Osteoporosis, *J Am Pharm Assoc* 44(2):152–60.

Grossberndt, S., van den Hazel, P., & Bartonova, A., 2012, Application of social media in the environment and health professional community, *Environ Health* Jun 28;11 (Suppl 1):S16.

Haddock, J., & Burrows, C., 1997, The role of the nurse in health promotion: an evaluation of a smoking-cessation programme in surgical pre-admission clinics, *J Adv Nurs* 26(6):1098–110.

Harris, M., Smith B., & Veale A., 2005, Printed patient education interventions to facilitate shared management of chronic disease: a literature review, *Intern Med J* 35(12):711–6.

Hearn, S., Nancarrow, H., Rose, M., Massi, L., Wise, M., Conigrave, K., Barnes, I., & Bauman, A., 2011, Evaluating NSW SmokeCheck: a culturally specific smoking cessation program for health professionals working in Aboriginal Health, *Health Promot J Aust* 22(3).

James, R., Tyler, C., Van Beurden, E., & Henrikson, D., 1989, Implementing a public cholesterol-screening campaign: the north coast experience, *Community Health Stud* 13(2):130–9.

Kirk, A., Mutrie, N., MacIntyre, P., & Fisher, M., 2003, Increasing physical activity in people with diabetes, *Diabet Care* 26(4):1186–92.

Kreuter, M.W., & McClure, S.M., 2004, The role of culture in health communication, *Annual Rev Public Health* 25:439–55.

Lawson, P.J., Flock, S.A., 2009, Teachable moments for health behavior change: a concept analysis, *Patient Educ Couns* 76(1):25–30.

Lorig, K.R., & Holman, H., 2003, Self-management education: history, definition, outcomes, and mechanisms, *Ann Behav Med* 26(1):1–7.

McMahon, S., 1990, Health promotion and cardiovascular risk factors, Paper presented to the Public Health Association Health Promotion Division Annual Meeting, Melbourne, Vic.

Medicare Locals, 2011, *Medicare Locals: Discussion paper on governance and functions*, Australian Government, Canberra, www.yourhealth.gov.au/internet/yourHealth/publishing.nsf/Content/MedicareLocalsDiscussionPaper/$FILE/Discussion%20Paper.pdf, accessed 10 April 2013.

Meyer, M., 2004, Physician use of email: the telephone of the 21st century?, *J Med Pract Manage* 19(5):247–51.

Miller, W.R., & Rollnick, S., 2002, *Motivational Interviewing*, Guilford Press, London.

Nuovo, J., Balsbaugh, T., Barton, S., Fong, R., Fox-Garcia, J., Levich, B., & Fenton, J.J., 2007, Interventions to support diabetes self-management: the key role of the patient in diabetes care, *Curr Diabet Rev* 3:226–8.

Nutbeam, D., 2009, Defining and measuring health literacy: what can we learn from literacy studies?, *Int J Public Health* 54(5):303–5.

Osborne, H., 2012, *Health Literacy: From A to Z*, Jones and Bartlett Learning, Burlington, Massachusetts.

Owen, N., 1988, Mediated instruction for smoking cessation: hooks, kits and audiovisual materials, in Byrne, D. (Ed.), *Smoking Behaviour and its Treatment*, ANU Press, Canberra.

Pai, C.W., Hagen, S.E., Bender, J., Shoemaker, D., & Edington, D.W., 2009, Effect of health risk appraisal frequency on change in health status, *J Occup Environ Med* Apr;51(4):429–34.

Pearson, C., & Seligman, M., 2004, *Character Strengths and Virtues*, Oxford University Press, US.

Ratzan, S.C., & Parker, R.M., 2000, Introduction, in Seldom, C.R., Zorn, M., Ratzan, S.C., et al. (Eds), *Current Bibliographies in Medicine: Health Literacy*, National Library of Medicine Pub. no. CBM 2000-1, National Institutes of Health, US Department of Health and Human Services, Washington, DC.

Redman, B.K., 2001, *Patient Education* (9th edn), C.V. Mosby, St Louis.

Richards, D., Toop, L., Brockway, K., Graham, S., McSweeney, B., MacLean, D., Sutherland, M., & Parsons, A., 2003, Improving the effectiveness of smoking cessation in primary care: lessons learned, *NZ Med J* 116:1173.

Richmond, R.L., Novak, K., Kehoe, L., Calfas, G., & Mendelsohn, C.P., 1998, Effect of training on general practitioners' use of a brief intervention for excessive drinkers, *Aust NZ J Public Health* 22:206–9.

Roberts, J., Browne G.B., Streiner, D., Gafni, A., Pallister, R., Hoxby H., Jamieson, E., & Meichenbaum, D., 1995, The effectiveness and efficiency of health promotion in specialty health clinic care, *Med Care* Sep;33(9):892–905.

Roland, M., & Dixon, M., 1989, Randomised controlled trial of an educational booklet for patients presenting with back pain in general practice, *J Royal College Gen Pract* (39):244–6.

Sherwood, N.E., Morton, N., Jeffery, R.W., French, S.A., Neumark-Sztainer, D., & Falkner, N.H., 1998, Consumer preferences in format and type of community-based weight control programs, *Am J Health Promot* 13(1):12–18.

Sinclair, H.K., Bond, C.M., & Stead, L.F., 2004, Community pharmacy personnel interventions for smoking cessation, *Cochrane Database Syst Rev* (1):CD003698.

Wallace, P., Cutler, A., & Haines, F., 1988, Randomised controlled trial of general practitioner intervention in patients with excessive alcohol consumption, *BMJ* 297:663–8.

Watkins, C.J., Papacosta, A.O., Chinn, S., & Martin, J.A., 1987, A randomised controlled trial of an information booklet for hypertensive patients in general practice, *J Royal College Gen Pract* 7:548–50.

WHO (World Health Organization), 1983, *Primary Health Care in Industrialised Countries: Report on the 1983 Conference in Bordeaux on Primary Health Care in Industrialized Countries*, WHO Euro Reports and Studies, WHO, Copenhagen.

chapter **4**

Focus on groups

Summary of main points

- Group processes can be a useful strategy on the continuum from one-to-one to population-level approaches.

- Health promotion in groups can be didactic, experiential or peer support, and the choice depends on circumstances as well as the intended audience.

- Group skills include an understanding of the processes of learning, group dynamics and communication.

- Most school-based and higher education occurs in groups.

- Group work can include 'train-the-trainer' options and capacity building to facilitate other health promotion strategies that are individual or population focused.

- Advances in interactive technology have expanded the possibilities for group work in health promotion.

- A new process of shared medical appointments (group visits) developed in the US might offer a new opportunity for managing chronic diseases in primary care.

Group processes in health promotion

If only on grounds of cost-effectiveness, individual strategies in health promotion are usually complemented by strategies reaching a wider audience. Group techniques offer an intermediate approach between one-to-one processes and wider, community-focused campaigns. The group process is not only a key modality for implementing health promotion programs, but it has also been used for many years by other professionals—such as adult education specialists, social workers and psychologists.

Groups can range in size from two or three people to a hundred or more, and can be *homogeneous* or *heterogeneous* in nature. Health promotion methods in such groups are classified here as *didactic* (e.g. lectures, seminars), *experiential* (e.g. skills training, role playing, simulation/games) or peer support related (e.g. special interest/ailment focused such as patient support groups). This classification is somewhat arbitrary, and others use a range of different classifications (e.g. see Johnson & Johnson 2012; Corey, Corey & Corey 2008; Corey 2003). In line with the rationale of this book, our dichotomy puts the emphasis on *process* rather than on *content, setting* or *program*. The didactic method emphasises, but is not restricted to, persuasion or knowledge transmission ('predisposing' factors), whereas the experiential approach emphasises skills training ('enabling' factors—see Green & Kreuter 2004). Peer support groups are usually self-generated and based around a particularly intractable ailment (e.g. asthma, chronic obstructive pulmonary disease, diabetes). An interesting new use of the peer support approach is through shared medical appointments or group visits within the primary care environment. These are discussed towards the end of this chapter.

A fourth use of groups in health promotion is as a source of information. *Focus groups*, for example, can be used in formative research (Krueger & Casey 2008; Stewart, Shamdasani & Rook 2006). In contrast to didactic and experiential approaches, which are used primarily to impart information to group participants, focus groups are used to gain information from participants, which can be used to help structure later health promotion initiatives. Finally, groups can also be for end-users (patients) or primary care workers to help them improve their management skills.

The ultimate goal of group methods as used by health promotion practitioners is to empower individuals, organisations and communities by:

- assisting individuals to modify or maintain health-related behaviours
- providing a supportive setting for individuals sharing a common goal or problem
- organising community or organisational members to improve their capacity to identify and solve their own problems (i.e. capacity building or community organisation)
- organising individuals and groups to undertake macro-level social change (e.g. training community leaders, coalition building)
- developing personal health and peer support programs in schools.

And in the case of focus groups, by:

- helping health promotion practitioners more accurately plan programs.

Group methods can be used in a range of different settings, classified by the level of prevention:

- *primary prevention*—including schools, workplaces and organisations

- *secondary prevention*—including medical practices, community health centres, outpatient clinics and drug-referral centres
- *tertiary prevention*—including hospitals, rehabilitation centres and nursing homes.

Modern technology (i.e. the internet) has enabled the ability to form a group from geographically dispersed, disparate individuals around issues of common interest and concern, unlike earlier days when a notice on a wall called people to a community hall or a room in a town square.

What is a group?

For health promotion application, Loomis's (1979) definition of a group still applies:

> A group is a collection of individuals who are to some degree interdependent. Within this definition, a number of people waiting for the elevator do not constitute a group. If that same collection of individuals needs to decide whether or not they will allow smoking on the elevator, then they become a group for the purpose of making that decision. Their common task has made them interdependent and therefore a group.

Group behaviour in the influence process has been studied for some time—paralleling the growth of group psychotherapy processes begun by the early psychoanalysts in the 1920s and 30s. In the 1960s—an era of unprecedented growth in the study of interpersonal relations and personal awareness—these two lines of development converged. The differences between group processes for the sick and learning practices for the well were broken down and the cross-cultivation of skills emerged. Since that time, groups have become applied to just about every health-related issue, from losing weight to learning natural childbirth (see box on page 108–9 for a list of self-help groups). Group processes have also become a study in themselves, with many contemporary exponents (e.g. see Corey, Corey & Corey 2008; Cragan, Wright & Kasch 2008; Johnson & Johnson 2012).

Group dynamics

Group dynamics is the study of the nature and development of groups and the interrelationship of group members with each other and other organisations. Group process skills are relevant in experiential situations, but are of less relevance in the didactic (e.g. lecturing) situation. Research on group dynamics has described groups in terms of the leadership, membership, goals, norms and interaction of group members (Cragan, Wright & Kasch 2008).

The characteristics of group communication include the following.

- *Group communication occurs in a system*—this implies that there is a connection between all dimensions involved. The dominance of any one dimension (e.g. leadership, membership) may vary in different types of groups, but ultimately it is the system that is affected by changes.
- *Group communication dimensions are simultaneously cause and effect*— a message may affect, or be affected by, components of the group system—depending on other characteristics of the group.
- *Group communication is dynamic*—changes that occur in groups are continuous, irreversible and unrepeatable, and the group facilitator must be aware of this in using the group process.
- *Group communication is complex*—any reduction of the group process to simple unidimensional factors will lead to conclusions on behalf of the facilitator that may be counterproductive in the group process. Group processes, unlike the didactic process, are complex and variable.

Group methods

Each of the different approaches to group health promotion listed below calls for different expertise—and no single health promotion practitioner may be expert in all. The didactic approach, for example, calls for content knowledge, lecturing skills and the ability to answer questions clearly. The experiential approach demands a sensitivity to and awareness of group processes. Qualitative research groups require a different set of skills based on questioning, listening and interpreting. Naturally, there is overlap between approaches: lectures and seminars, for example, are usually more effective when there is two-way interaction between presenter and audience. Similarly, experiential learning can benefit from the high content knowledge of a group leader.

The didactic method is commonly used when the goal is transmission of knowledge or information. Lectures on chronic disease, for instance, might have as their goal the simple transmission of information about chronic disease risk and risk factor behaviours. As such, the didactic approach is generally individualistic—that is, directed at groups of individuals to bring about individual behaviour change. There are occasions, however, when the didactic method may be used to stimulate actions to influence more collective actions such as socio-environmental changes, which may relate more to the social determinants of health—for example, information-based lectures on the environment and climate change or on social inequities.

Experiential group learning is perhaps best performed when the behavioural outcome required is a complex one and requires the detailed development of components identified in health behaviour theory models

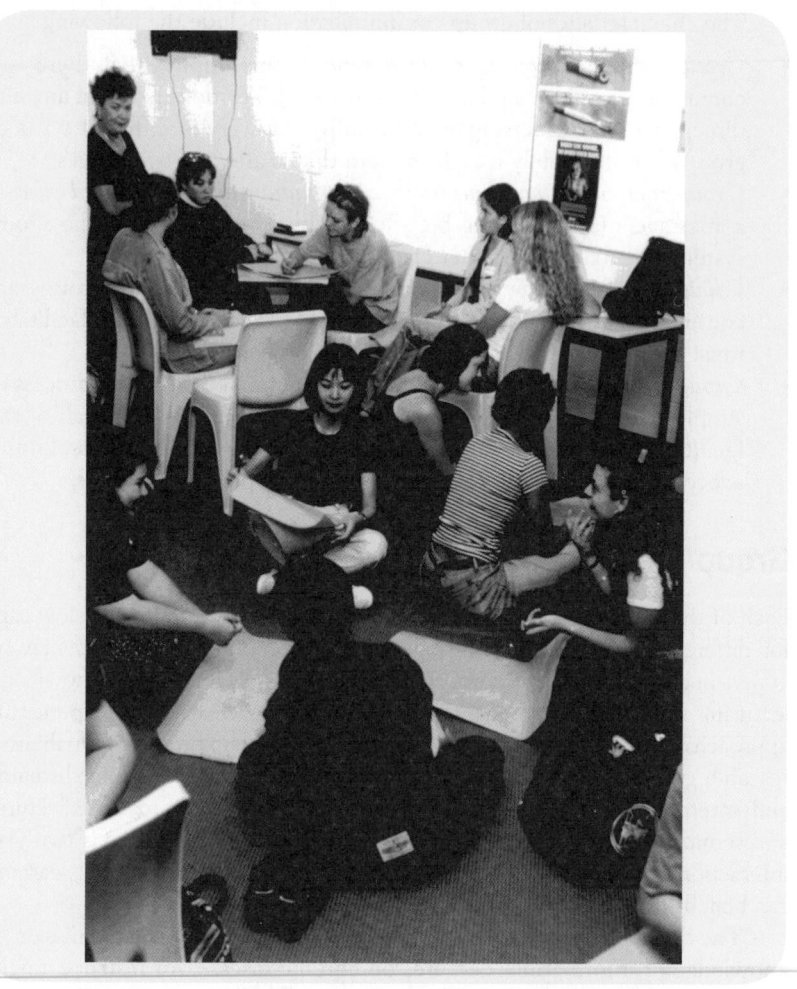

Groups held as part of motivational seminars on nutrition, fitness, self-esteem, drug use and job preparation conducted for young female school leavers by the Smoking and Health Team

Health Department of Western Australia

as influencing behaviour—that is, intentions, attitudes, barriers and beliefs (see Chapter 2).

The predisposing effect of knowledge, attitudes and beliefs about chronic disease (perceived susceptibility) gained from didactic and other methods can be used to motivate individuals to practise and learn skills (enabling factors) in the experiential situation.

CASE STUDY **4.1**

'Edu-venture' workshops for health and medical professionals

Continuing professional development (CPD) is an important part of postgraduate training in many professional spheres, particularly those in which there is rapidly changing information, such as medicine and the health sciences. Because much modern chronic disease is caused by lifestyle, it seems inappropriate to teach the new field of 'lifestyle medicine' (e.g. see www.lifestylemedicine.com.au) in a classroom.

Southern Cross University in New South Wales, in conjunction with the Australian Lifestyle Medicine Association, is the first tertiary institution to conduct lifestyle medicine training through a process called 'edu-ventures'. Doctors and allied health professionals are taken on 4–7-day trips, paddling, bush or desert walking, or carrying out other outdoor activities during the daytime, while experiencing a variety of short CPD courses during the day and in the evenings. The group and peer support processes during the activities help add to the lectures and interactive learning sessions, while providing a holiday and necessary CPD points for ongoing professional accreditation.

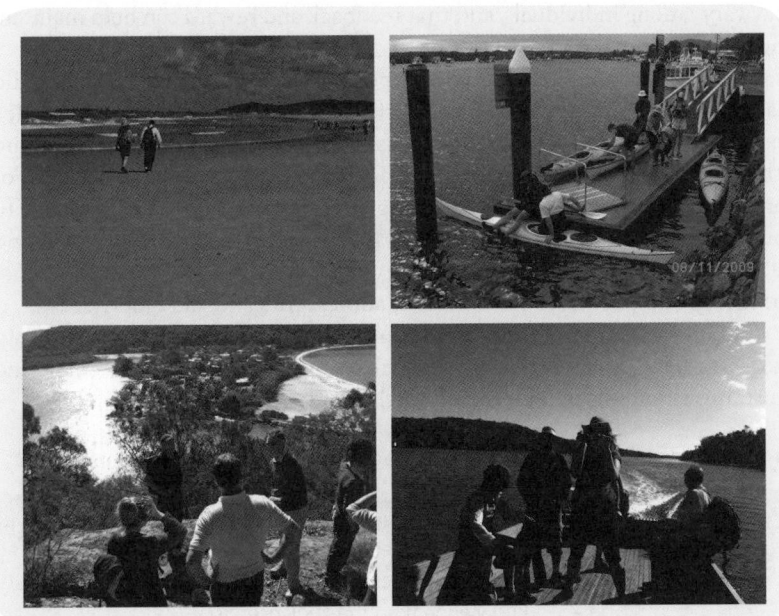

Doctors and health professionals during various 'edu-ventures'

Australian Lifestyle Medicine Association (www.lifestylemedicine.com.au)

Adult learning

The education of adults, as opposed to children and adolescents, is a multifaceted, complex process that encompasses many subject and interest areas. There has been a whole area of study devoted to the topic over the last 30 years (e.g. see Verduin, Miller & Greer 1979). Because adults have lived for and experienced a given number of years, they have had the opportunity to gain many perceptions of their environment and the objects and events in it. An adult's past experience then forms the basis from which education and behaviour change must commence. Adult behaviour at this stage may be more rigid than that of younger people because adult behaviour has been formed over a longer period of time.

Since the modification of perception and behaviour in adult groups is personal and requires attention to threat processing, any adult learning program should be as individual as possible. This requires keeping the individual moving towards his or her goal. Since retention may be a problem in adult learning situations, it is important to emphasise progress and to continually reinforce learned practices.

Lack of progress in achieving goals among some adult learners can be attributed to low self-esteem and a lack of self-confidence. Facilitators/ trainers need to take account of this, as well as the fact that learning rates may vary among individuals, and that feedback and reward can help maintain and enhance motivation.

Finally, since adult learning may be a more gradual process than child learning, adults must be given appropriate time and guidance to experience and develop new behaviours. Some tasks may take more time to learn and others less—illustrating again the importance of individual attention. For further information on adult learning principles, readers are referred to sources such as Knowles, Swanson & Hotlon (2011), Rothwell (2008) and Tate (2012). Other authors (e.g. Corey, Corey & Corey 2008) also discuss specific group processes for children, adolescents and the elderly.

Table 4.1 is a summary of the methods and characteristics of group processes. The discussion that follows explains the processes in detail and illustrates situations in which each might be best utilised.

Table 4.1: A summary of group methods in health promotion

Didactic group methods	
Lecture–discussion	Best for knowledge transmission, motivation in large groups. Requires dynamic, effective speaker with more knowledge than the audience.
Seminar	Smaller numbers (2–20). Leader–group feedback. Leader most knowledgeable in the group. Best for trainer learning.

Conference	Larger numbers (50–5000). Can combine lecture/ seminar techniques. Best for professional development.
Videoconferencing	Opportunity for group learning for professionals such as rural and remote doctors and nurses.
Web-based seminars/ discussions (webinars)	Generally didactic but can provide opportunity for interaction.
Experiential group methods	
Skills training	Requires motivated individuals. Includes explanation, demonstration and practice, for example, relaxation, childbirth, exercise.
Behaviour modification	Learning and unlearning of specific habits. Stimulus–response learning. Generally behaviour-specific, for example, smoking cessation, phobia desensitisation.
Enquiry learning	Used mainly in school settings. Requires formulating and problem solving through group cooperation.
Peer group discussion	Useful where shared experiences, support and awareness are important. Participants homogeneous in at least one factor, for example, old people, prisoners, teenagers.
Simulation	Useful for influencing attitudes in individuals with varying abilities. Generally in school setting, but of relevance to other groups.
Role play	Acting of roles by group participants. Can be useful where communication difficulties exist between individuals in a setting, for example, families, professional practice. Requires skilled facilitator.
Self-help	Requires motivation and independent attitude. Valuable for ongoing peer support, values clarification. Can be therapy or a forum for social action.
Shared medical appointments (SMAs)	A process for dealing with chronic disease in the primary care situation involving GPs and other allied health professionals in a group medical consultation (see p. 106).

Detailed explanation of methods

Didactic methods

Didactic approaches involve the health promotion practitioner in a predominantly authoritative role with an audience or individual. There are a number of different ways of doing this.

Lecture–discussion

The lecture, presentation or talk is one of the oldest teaching methods around. Recourse to any historical science book will relate numerous circumstances of seminal lectures—the date, time, place and topic—delivered by now revered thinkers who have had a role in changing the world.[1] As a health education practice, however, the lecture–discussion is one of the most difficult to master. Part of the professional process of health promotion practitioners is to be aware of their skills and limitations. If a lecture situation is required, and the practitioner does not have the necessary skills, he or she should attempt to develop these—or facilitate other professionals with the appropriate skills. Groups such as Toastmasters and other organisations and associations can help develop these skills.

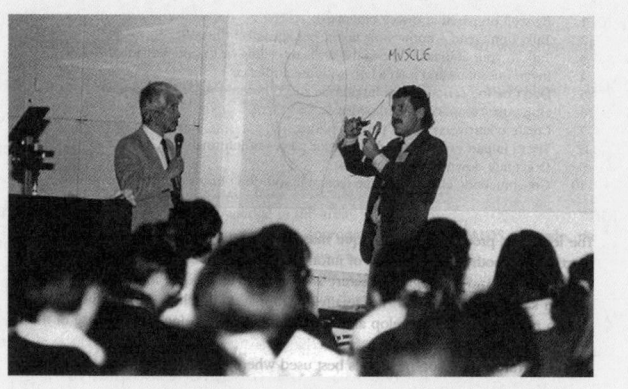

The lecture is a longstanding method of health promotion

The advantages of the lecture are that it is easy to use, can impart information, can influence opinion and can stimulate thought and critical thinking. Lectures are economical and practical, and can incorporate dialogue between lecturer and participants. The disadvantages are that lecturing involves skills that may be difficult for the lecturer to master, the audience is generally passive (and therefore less likely to learn in some cases), and the lecture approach is not suited to the learning of complex skills.

Some of the world's leading exponents of the didactic approach are now seen on websites such as www.ted.com, where speakers are given limited time to get a view across to a worldwide audience. (For an excellent example discussing the problem with the modern Western diet in 3 minutes and 22 seconds, see www.ted.com/talks/dean_ornish_on_the_world_s_killer_diet.html.) Didactic seminars can also be catalysts for generating new ideas, such as the annual Festival of Dangerous Ideas in Sydney.

The efficacy of the lecture as a means of education is unquestioned. What is less certain, however, is the comparative effectiveness of the lecture in contrast to other techniques (e.g. discussion groups, educational films, video). Indeed, each technique has its advantages under different conditions. Research carried out by Green as long ago as 1978 found that the lecture is less effective than group discussion and other methods where there is a need for attitudinal change or the development of problem-solving or values-clarification skills. It is also probable that the didactic approach works differently for different audiences. Table 4.1 discusses use of the lecture approach with doctors, who because of their objective training in physiological information and their cognitive ability respond well to this approach.

The lecture is probably the most used technique by health educators and other health practitioners, both for transmission of information to the public and training of professional groups. Although the lecture is a valuable technique, it may be overused and used in situations where it is not totally appropriate. The challenge for the health promotion practitioner is to develop an educational mix, which includes the use of the lecture in appropriate situations.

Tips for planning a good lecture

1. Know your subject—or at least that part of it about which you are going to speak.
2. Prepare audiovisuals to accompany your main points.
3. Speak slowly and clearly—use a microphone if more than a few people.
4. Make eye contact with the audience.
5. Always look at the audience—don't talk to the screen.
6. Plan your timing closely—avoid the no. 1 sin: going overtime.
7. Don't go too slow at the start and then have to speed up to get the main points in.
8. Tell them what you're going to tell them; tell them; then tell them what you told them.
9. Never admit to the audience that you are nervous or scared!
10. Remember, it takes a lifetime for someone to find out what you know, but only one sentence to find out what you don't!

If using a computer-generated visual presentation (e.g. PowerPoint):

- present issues one at a time
- make the best use of colour
- make use of contrast in colours
- don't put too much on one screen
- consider short videos embedded in the presentation if these make a point
- use fewer slides rather than too many
- use the computer-generated presentation as an adjunct to your presentation, not as the presentation itself.

The lecture–discussion method is appropriate when:

- information transmission and motivation are the main goals
- the lecturer knows more than the group about the subject
- the group is too large for small group activity
- all participants need to hear the same information in the same way
- the lecturer is a dynamic, informative and sensitive speaker
- the audience is reasonably motivated and aware of and interested in the topic.

Seminar/workshop

The seminar involves elements of the lecture–discussion approach with more group interaction. Generally, the numbers involved are smaller (2 to 15), allowing greater interaction with the seminar leader.

The main difference between the seminar and the experiential technique is that seminars are generally more information based, rather than skills based, and involve some didactic discussion from a leader with greater knowledge of content than the group. Seminars are most effective in training of trainers or other health professionals, where it is important for the leader to get feedback about learning from the group. The seminar method is most appropriate when:

- small numbers are involved
- lecturer–participant feedback is important
- groups are homogeneous (e.g. diabetics, asthmatics, nurses)
- there are limitations of space and time
- professional training is required
- the seminar leader knows more about the topic than the group.

Conference

A conference is usually a combination of the lecture and seminar/workshop techniques. It is usually reserved for professional development and networking and is generally conducted over several hours or days. The conference usually requires several 'keynote' authorities in the subject areas, and can be conducted with large groups of people (in large and smaller groups). Conference delegates usually get their own opportunity to present information or research via proffered papers, often to smaller audiences, depending on the overall number of people attending the conference. Conferences are generally specific to a topic or subject area or theme. The method is appropriate when:

- professional updating of information is required
- several experts in the field can be involved
- there is a need for consensus among professionals
- participants have basic knowledge in the area.

Webinars or web-based seminars

The rapid spread of the internet has led to the development of web-based seminars or webinars, where participants can interact from any part of the world. These are used increasingly in tertiary education and as postgraduate training for professionals in rural and remote areas in particular. Webinars are useful when:

- there is a wide geographical spread
- participants would find it difficult to attend in person
- after-hours attendance is feasible, possible and preferred
- the material can be accessed in 'real time' or recorded for later use.

Suitability for the didactic approach

Appropriate subjects for the didactic approach include lectures on:

- HIV/AIDS
- lifestyle
- risk factors
- parenthood
- infant health
- nutrition
- exercise
- immunisation.

Less appropriate situations for the didactic approach include:

- community development
- stress management
- quit-smoking training
- drug therapy
- mental health
- family therapy
- weight control
- peer support programs.

CASE STUDY **4.2**

Preventing scalds in New Zealand school children

A school-based scalds prevention program for school groups involving just two classroom sessions and a homework exercise that targeted five safety practices shows the value of this type of education long term.

The program was taught to 28 classes in 14 schools in Waitakere City, New Zealand, by public health nurses (PHNs). Children aged 10–11 years from three of the schools in ethnically diverse, low and middle-income areas were then assessed for their knowledge of scalds hazards one year after the program.

They recalled a mean of 7.46 out of 10 hazards. Altogether, 65–79 per cent of children reported that each of the five safety practices provided were at least temporarily used as intended, with 29–55 per cent reporting that they were still in use one year later. Interviews with children's parents indicated that the majority of their hot water practices were not optimally safe prior to the program and that many had adopted the suggested practices. While the PHNs were positive about the program, they suggested teachers could also deliver it as part of the school curriculum.

Moore, Morath & Harre 2004

Experiential methods

> I hear and I forget. I see and I remember. I do and I understand.
>
> —Confucius

Working with small groups

Working with groups is a key role of the health promotion practitioner, whether they be *focus groups* (in needs assessment and planning), *discussion groups* (for education and awareness-raising) or *learning groups* (for behaviour modification skills training).

In some respects, small groups as used in health promotion are similar to processes involved in focus group interviews. The focus group interview is a qualitative research technique used to obtain data about perceptions, feelings and opinions of small groups of participants about a given problem, experience, service, product or other phenomenon. Focus group research is concerned with eliciting and understanding concepts rather than with measuring them—for example, expanding knowledge, identifying and clarifying issues, identifying behaviours, explaining behaviours, generating hypotheses and providing input into future research.

Characteristics of small groups as used in health promotion are as follows:

* the size of the group is usually 6–12 people (although this is flexible, and productive sessions can be conducted with fewer or more participants)
* discussions usually last 1–3 hours
* a 'safe' or non-threatening setting (physically and psychologically) is required
* the group leader or facilitator requires skill in facilitating effective communication, and is of key importance to successful outcomes
* concerns, experiences and motives may be the subject of discussions.

Tactics of the group facilitator

Interpersonal tactics useful in the group situation include the following:

- *Be non-judgmental*—if group members feel that their opinions, attitudes and behaviours are likely to be judged as good or bad by the facilitator, they are less likely to contribute openly. This does not always mean agreeing with the attitudes and behaviours of others, but it does mean acceptance of differences.
- *Be honest*—sharing thoughts and feelings with a group is important in developing an open and trusting atmosphere. A willingness to do so by the facilitator can be a catalyst for others to contribute.
- *Foster trust*—this is an ongoing development that depends on the feedback that the group members receive from each other and the facilitator. If they feel accepted as worthwhile members of the group, trust in the group will develop.
- *Observe*—the facilitator needs to be a sensitive observer of the interactions, behaviours and underlying processes occurring in the group. If direction is lost, or the task becomes confused, it is up to the facilitator to get the group back on track with as little disruption as possible.
- *Be sensitive*—group members may sometimes share personal experiences that are personal and important to them. The facilitator needs to be sensitive to individuals' needs in order to aid the total group process.
- *Communicate*—effective communication is both verbal and non-verbal. In some situations (e.g. focus groups), it is important for facilitators to stay quiet so that their ideas do not influence the needs-assessment process. However, non-verbal cues—such as head nodding and shrugging—may be just as potent. Communication means listening, not just to words, but also tuning in on the other person's feelings. Effective communication by the facilitator will establish the opportunity for all to contribute and to feel valued as group members.
- *Be flexible*—leadership styles vary according to the nature of a group and the stage of the group's development. For example, early in a group's life, more structure and direction may be required. As the group develops, the tasks may be developed and relationships in the group maintained with little direction from the facilitator.
- *Be firm*—it is inevitable that occasions will arise when group members display behaviour that may be disruptive to the group. Aggression, dominance of the discussions and other disruptive behaviours can cause others to become defensive, withdrawn or frustrated by the group's interaction. If left unchecked by the facilitator, these behaviours can result in a dysfunctional group.
- *Take account of varying health literacy levels*—it's a common mistake to think that everyone understands what is being communicated just

because no questions are asked. Techniques like 'teach back' (i.e. asking questions to make sure the participants understand) can help this process.

Skills training

This involves the group learning of skills that can facilitate the health process—for example, stress management, healthy cooking, prenatal breathing and self-care. The skill development method should provide explanation about the need for a procedure, demonstration of the procedure for the group, and practical experience in the procedure (Johnson & Johnson 2012).

Skills development can include training in communication for conflict resolution, self-assertion and group decision making. The procedure has been used in school health education programs to teach adolescents how to cope with peer pressure to smoke or take drugs (Rohsenhow & Monti 2012). Computer software programs have been developed to assist young people in the development of life skills. For example, SMART Talk—a multimedia, computer-based, violence prevention intervention—employs games, simulations, graphics, cartoons and interactive interviews to engage young adolescents in learning new skills to resolve conflicts without violence (Bosworth et al. 1996).

Skills training is most effective when techniques are required for 'coping' with situations that may be adverse to health. It should be used only with participants whose values and intentions have been clearly defined.

Health promotion practitioners utilising small group methods frequently within their roles may benefit from formal training in group facilitation techniques available from reputable training organisations in most capital cities and some regional centres. Certain group topics—such as stress management, interpersonal communication skills training, role play and exercise instruction—are a useful addition to any health promoter's armoury. These can be learned from a number of sources (e.g. Johnson & Johnson 2012). For other, more specific skills training, the practitioner can draw on specialist expertise such as that of counsellors and psychologists.

Behaviour modification

As described in Chapter 2, behaviour modification is the specific process of learning and unlearning habits based on stimulus–response learning theory. The process requires the facilitator to have skills, knowledge and an understanding of learning theory principles, such as reinforcement (anything that increases a response), punishment (anything that decreases a response), stimulus generalisation (responding to cues that are similar to the originally conditioned cue), and extinction (when a response ceases because it is no longer reinforced).Behaviour modification can be carried out in groups or individually and is generally used to unlearn unhealthy habits, although the method can be used to develop healthy habits as a component of other health promotion programs—such as exercise. Behaviour modification is most suited to situations that involve individuals who are motivated and informed but have difficulty breaking old habits (Simon-Morton, McLeroy & Wendel 2011). Examples include quit smoking, weight control, diet and anxiety reduction programs.

Enquiry learning

Enquiry learning was developed under the patronage of psychologist Jerome Bruner (1966). In this process, often used in schools, group participants are encouraged to formulate and test their own hypotheses—which they can do in small groups, through practical excursions, reading and personal experience.

CASE STUDY 4.3

School groups, soft drink consumption and health promotion practice

As with any new claim against vested interests in health, the first stage is often one of denial or the claim that there is 'no convincing evidence' of a connection between a manufacturer's product and ill-health. Reaction from the tobacco industry against claims initially made in 1950 continued in this fashion for 3–4 decades, despite over 50 000 research articles proving a link between smoking and cancer. More recently, a link between soft drink consumption and obesity was found by British researchers. They found a reduction in soft drink use and weight loss in children from schools where group education about the risks of soft drink use was carried out, compared to control schools where this did not occur. This is likely to increase demands on soft drink control as a public health measure.

James et al. 2004

The enquiry learning approach is applicable to some community group settings—for example, patient–doctor interactions—although it is not often used by health promotion practitioners.

Peer group discussion/support

Discussion methods are often regarded as superior to the lecture method where a homogeneous group with a common purpose exists. In schools, discussion is often practised to develop an understanding and awareness of the processes of peer pressure involved in many health-associated behaviours (e.g. drinking, drug-taking, sexual activity). Peer groups are useful for shared experiences, group support, awareness raising and idea generation. Peer education programs have also been employed successfully in the delivery of health education programs for high-risk populations such as those at high risk for HIV/AIDS. With a skilful leader, groups such as senior citizens, prisoners, patients and students can benefit from the peer group discussion–interaction process. The technique also involves processes included in other group methods (i.e. sensitivity groups and role play).

The introduction of the internet and chat groups has made the discussion method a popular one for widespread group involvement with people who have something in common. No doubt many more opportunities will develop in this area as the technology expands.

Shared medical appointments

Shared medical appointments (SMAs) (group visits) are a new and innovative way of dealing with chronic diseases in primary care. Traditionally, management of disease has been done one-to-one in a clinical situation. While this has served us well (and still does) for infectious diseases and injury, it appears less appropriate for chronic diseases, which require longer-term management. Because most chronic diseases have a limited number of lifestyle-related causes, sufferers from many different kinds of problems (e.g. heart disease, diabetes, cancers, respiratory problems) can benefit from the experience of others as well as the help of health professionals.

SMAs were developed in the US in the 1990s, and have been broadened to include several different forms, such as Drop-In Group Medical Appointments (DIGMAs) and physical shared medical appointments. The approach has been defined as '*comprehensive medical visits (billable at individual rates) focusing on chronic disease, but run in a supportive group setting of consenting patients with similar concerns, and run with 2–4 appropriate health professionals, including a GP*' (Noffsinger 2009). Several textbooks and articles have now been written on the process (Noffsinger 2009, 2012; Berger-Fiffy 2012), although the process has not yet been utilised in Australia.

SMAs offer the advantage of cutting down waiting times in primary care, utilising peer support, having a full medical assessment involving a variety of health professionals and reducing healthcare costs. In a world of changing disease prevalence, the process may help provide a solution to the modern healthcare dilemma. Confidentiality agreements need to be drawn up, however, and individuals will need to become familiar with a new form of healthcare and health promotion delivery.

Simulation

Simulation refers to the process of enacting a real-life experience. Simulation learning in groups can take the form of games, dramatisation, role play, case studies and repeats of actual experience. Where simulations are carried out, group leaders should be well prepared, know the outcome of the process and be ready for appropriate actions and questions.

Because of their nature as games, simulations with health education intent have usually been confined to the classroom. However, with the rapid advancement of computer technologies, there is increasing scope for the development of computer-based games and simulations that have application to health promotion. For example, Johnston and colleagues (2012) investigated an alternative reality game as a means to influence college students' physical activity towards reducing obesity risk. They found a significant increase in physical activity for the game group over the comparison group and concluded that there is evidence that a game can positively influence physical activity, at least within a college student population.

Also in terms of the promotion of physical activity, the advent of active video games (AVGs) provides the tempting scenario where individuals, the family or neighbourhood group can potentially become active instead of sedentary thanks to modern technology. In a systematic review of the current state of research into AVGs for physical activity promotion, Peng and colleagues (2012) concluded that AVGs are capable of providing light-to-modest physical activity for both children and adults. However, little support was found for the long-term efficacy of using AVGs in a non-structured and self-managed manner for physical activity promotion. These researchers suggested that it may be more promising to employ AVGs in a structured exercise program in a group setting and noted that specifically designed AVGs guided by behaviour-change theories are needed.

Social networking websites such as Facebook and MySpace provide not only opportunities for increased social interactivity but also health promotion potential. However these sites can be limited in that they can only process pieces of information consecutively and even instant messaging lacks a physical presence for communication exchange. Cowdrey and colleagues (2011) successfully utilised the online virtual world Second Life (www.secondlife.com) for the delivery of health promotion messages (via a health educator 'avatar') to encourage a group of students to make healthy lifestyle choices regarding physical activity and nutrition. Because of the enhanced feeling of 'presence' experienced by participants, the use of virtual worlds in health-related applications, including health promotion, is likely to be explored more fully in the future.

Role play

Role play involves acting out an experience in the way an individual would enact that behaviour. For example, it may involve teenagers in a group talking like the smoker of a particular advertised brand of cigarettes, or adults acting the problems of a drug user in order to understand the problems of that individual.

Role play can be structured (preplanned, rehearsed) or unstructured (impromptu). There are five techniques that help the role play situation:

- *role reversal*—where individuals mimic each other
- *soliloquy*—where the actors are asked about their feelings
- *doubling*—where observers interject their feelings
- *multiple role playing*—where several participants act each role
- *role rotation*—where roles are changed during the action.

Role playing is most useful in the school situation, where people have difficulty expressing their thoughts about each other (e.g. in family education), and where roles are a significant hindrance to the health process (Bastable et al. 2010).

Self-help groups

Self-help has been discussed as an individual process in Chapter 3. Self-help groups now also exist in a range of different health-related areas (e.g. alcohol/drug abuse, domestic violence, weight control, gambling, parenthood, child abuse, and infectious and chronic diseases), both geographically and through the internet. Often these carry the epithet '– Anonymous' (e.g. 'Alcoholics Anonymous', 'Gamblers Anonymous', 'Over-eaters Anonymous') to encourage greater participation among those concerned about revealing their identity. The role of the health promotion practitioner is to facilitate and selectively recommend such groups, rather than become involved in the group process as such, which would defeat the main purpose of the group— that is, to develop self-esteem through individual and group action. Self-help groups can have therapy as their main purpose (e.g. drug abuse) or can be community and action-orientated (e.g. neighbourhood watch).

Men's Sheds are an example of an innovative approach to men's health: they get men involved more in their own health by tapping into their underlying interests, such as tool making, cars and building (see www.mensheds.org.au).

Self-help groups available on the internet

The rise of the internet has led to a huge increase in the number of self-help groups with immediate access to information on their ailment/condition. In many cases of obscure diseases, this has made patients greater experts than their doctors, and challenges the one-way education process from patient to doctor. Some relevant self-help group sites for prevalent modern disease categories include the following:

- Asthma, www.asthma.org.au
- Arthritis, www.arthritisaustralia.com.au
- Diabetes, www.diabetesincontrol.com
- Depression, www.beyondblue.org.au

- General self-help advice/support groups, www.healthinsite.gov.au (Aust. Government)
- Heartburn (reflux), www.nlm.nih.gov/medlineplus/gerd.html
- Pregnancy, www.mydr.com.au/search/support-groups?q=pregnancy%20and%20 childbirth
- Sleep disorders, www.sleepoz.org.au
- Weight control, www.anzos.com

This list is non-exhaustive and websites may change over time. Readers are advised to use an internet search engine to seek out contemporary groups.

Suitability for experiential approach

Appropriate situations for the experiential approach include:

- behaviour learning
- risk factor modification
- interpersonal skills
- substance abuse
- self-care
- quit smoking exercises
- weight control
- family education
- sex education
- coping skills and self-esteem training
- personal hygiene
- family planning
- healthy cooking classes.

Less appropriate situations for the experiential approach include:

- infectious disease information
- immunisation education.

Some practicalities in conducting group methods

Most people wishing to develop group learning activities assume that an army of paid group leaders on significant salaries is a basic requirement. Such an approach is obviously economically impractical. There are, however, effective alternatives using the principles that have been developed in marketing. The essential features are:

- the participants pay
- the income is used to employ group leaders
- group leaders can be recruited from successful former group-participants who then receive formal training in group facilitation.

Allowances can be made for free participation by low-income earners.

There are many successful examples of this approach with literally thousands of participants from both affluent and less affluent neighbourhoods creating and running groups on topics such as child rearing, stress reduction and weight control. A highly successful example of this technique, which has become a commercial venture, is Weight Watchers International (see Case study 4.4).

CASE STUDY **4.4**

Weight loss in groups: the Weight Watchers model

Weight Watchers was started in the 1960s initially for women to provide group support for fellow women faced with the onerous (and lonely) task of losing weight. The Weight Watchers approach has served as a model for weight control programs ever since. In the process, Weight Watchers has become a multinational organisation with shares on international stock markets. Despite several attempts to broaden the concept to males, its client base remains largely female, probably because of the nature of the group support provided, which has more appeal to women. Although commercially sensitive about its results, like most commercial weight loss programs, limited published data suggest that the program is more effective than self-help in achieving and maintaining weight loss in women.

Heshka et al. 2000

Summary of group methods

The focus on groups in this section has concentrated on practical skills useful for modifying health behaviour in a cost-effective manner. These techniques can satisfy the needs of dealing with high-risk individuals in the community but, in general, are likely to have little impact on the structural causes of ill-health.

The population-level approaches discussed in the next chapter extend the practitioner's ability to modify the health of individuals in a community, and introduce skills that also act on the social determinants of ill-health.

Career opportunities in health promotion

Career opportunities for health promotion professionals utilising group skills include teaching physical education/personal development in schools, or as a fitness or recreation officer in fitness and leisure centres, industry or the defence forces. Lecturing, either as a public or motivational speaker, or in an academic capacity, are other options. Opportunities also exist as a group moderator or facilitator, for example, as a diabetes, arthritis or asthma educator, either privately or for group medical or other practices and in such processes as shared medical appointments. Group leaders are often employed through private organisations such as adventure or personal development organisations or corporate health/ fitness programs. Audiovisual production and the development of web-based initiatives for specific group-based programs is another opportunity, given the increasing need to develop online programs such as for rural and remote health professionals. This can also include health professional, or 'train-the-trainer' options, such as teaching doctors, nurses, fitness leaders and other health specialists in lifestyle-based health, either face-to-face or in group situations.

Note

1. An excellent recent discussion of many of these is contained in Bill Bryson's popular book *A Short History of Nearly Everything* (2003, Broadway Books, USA).

References

Bastable, S., Gramet, P., Jacobs, K., & Sopczyk, D., 2010, *Health Professional as Educator: Principles of Teaching and Learning*, Jones and Bartlett Learning, Ontario.

Berger-Fiffy, J., 2012, The 'nuts and bolts' of implementing shared medical appointments, *J Ambul Care Manage* 35(3):247–56.

Bosworth, K., Espelage, D., DuBay, T., Dahlberg, L.L., & Daytner, G., 1996, Using multimedia to teach conflict-resolution skills to young adolescents, *Am J Prev Med* 12 (Suppl. 5):65–74.

Bruner, J.S., 1966, *Toward a Theory of Instruction*, Harvard University Press, Cambridge.

Corey, G., 2003, *Group Techniques* (3rd edn), Brooks/Cole, New York.

Corey, M.S., Corey, G., & Corey, C., 2008, *Groups: Process and Practice*, Brooks Cole, New York.

Cowdrey, J., Kindred, J., Michalakis, A., & Suggs, L., 2011, Promoting health in a virtual world: impressions of health communication messages delivered in second life, *First Monday* 16(9):23 August.

Cragan, J.F., Wright D.W., & Kasch, C.R., 2008, Communication in small groups: theory process and skills (with Infotrac), *The Wadsworth Series in Speech Communication* (10th edn), Wadsworth Publishing, London.

Green, L.W., 1978, Determining the impact and effectiveness of health education as it relates to federal policy, *Health Educ Monogr* 6(1):28–66.

Green, L.W., & Kreuter, M.W., 2004, *Health Promotion Planning: An Educational and Ecological Approach*, Mayfield Publishing Co., Mountain View.

Heshka, S., Greenway, F., Anderson, J. W., Atkinson, R. L., Hill, J. O., Phinney, S. D., Miller-Kovach, K., & Xavier Pi-Sunyer, F., 2000, Self-help weight loss versus a structured commercial program after 26 weeks: a randomized controlled study, *Am J Med* 109(4): 282–7.

James, J., Thomas, P., Cavan, D., & Kerr, D., 2004, Preventing childhood obesity by reducing consumption of carbonated drinks: cluster randomized controlled trial, *BMJ* 328(7450):1236.

Johnson, D.W., & Johnson, F.P, 2012, *Joining Together: Group Theory and Group Skills* (11th edn), Prentice-Hall, Englewood Cliffs.

Johnston, J. Massey, A., & Marker-Hoffman, R., 2012, Using an alternative reality game to increase physical activity and decrease obesity risk of college students, *J Diabetes Sci Technol* 6(4):828–38.

Knowles, M.S., Swanson, R.A., & Hotlon, E.F., 2011, *The Adult Learner, The Definitive Classic in Adult Education and Human Resource Development* (7th edn), Elsevier, Burlington, Massachusetts.

Krueger, RA., & Casey, M.A., 2008, *Focus Groups: A Practical Guide for Applied Research* (5th edn), Sage Publications, Thousand Oaks, California.

Loomis, M.E., 1979, *Group Processes for Nurses*, The C.V. Moseby Company, St. Louis.

Moore, J., Morath, K., & Harre, N., 2004, Follow-up study of a school-based scalds prevention programme, *Health Educ Res* 19(4):430–9.

Noffsinger, E., 2009, *Running Group Visits in Your Practice*, Springer, London.

Noffsinger, E., 2012, *The ABC of Group Visits*, Springer, London.

Peng, W., Crouse, J., & Jih-Hsuan, L, 2012, Using active video games for physical activity promotion: a systematic review of the current state of research, *Health Educ Behav* Jul 6:1–22.

Rohsenhow, D.J., & Monti, P.M., 2012, *Coping-Skills Training and Cue-Exposure Therapy in the Treatment of Alcoholism*, Department of Health and Human Services, US.

Rothwell, W.J., 2008, *Adult Learning Basics*, ASTD Training Basics Series, ASTD Press, Danvers, Massachusetts.

Simon-Morton, B., McLeroy, K.R., & Wendel M.L., 2011, *Behavior Theory in Health Promotion Practice and Research*, Jones and Bartlett, Burlington, Massachusetts.

Stewart, D.W., Shamdasani, P.N., & Rook, D., 2006, *Focus Groups: Theory and Practice (Applied Social Research Methods)*, Sage Publications, California.

Tate, M.L., 2012, *'Sit and Get' Won't Grow Dendrites: 20 Professional Learning Strategies That Engage the Adult Brain*, Sage, Thousand Oaks, California.

Verduin, J.R., Miller, H.G., & Greer, C.E, 1979, *Adults Teaching Adults*, Learning Concepts, Houston.

chapter **5**

Focus on populations:
social marketing

Summary of main points

- Social marketing is the application of commercial marketing techniques to the achievement of socially desirable goals.

- Marketing—and hence social marketing—is much more than just advertising; it is a comprehensive, integrated, multifaceted approach.

- Marketing is distinguished by a consumer orientation, and hence social marketing relies on research to identify, understand, reach and motivate the target audience, whether that be individuals in the general population, bureaucrats, manufacturers, marketers or policy makers.

- Social marketing targets individuals to modify their risky behaviours and targets individuals with power to modify the environment to facilitate individual behaviour change and risk reduction.

- Social marketing for health combines the principles of marketing, the principles of the Ottawa Charter, and a public health approach.

Social marketing

According to Schwartz (1995), social marketing is a program planning process that promotes voluntary behaviour change on the basis of:

- offering benefits people want
- reducing barriers people face
- using persuasion, not just information.

The term 'social marketing' appears to have been used first by Kotler and Zaltman in 1971 to describe the application of the principles and methods of marketing to the achievement of socially desirable goals. Since then, the use of marketing techniques in the health area has grown rapidly in

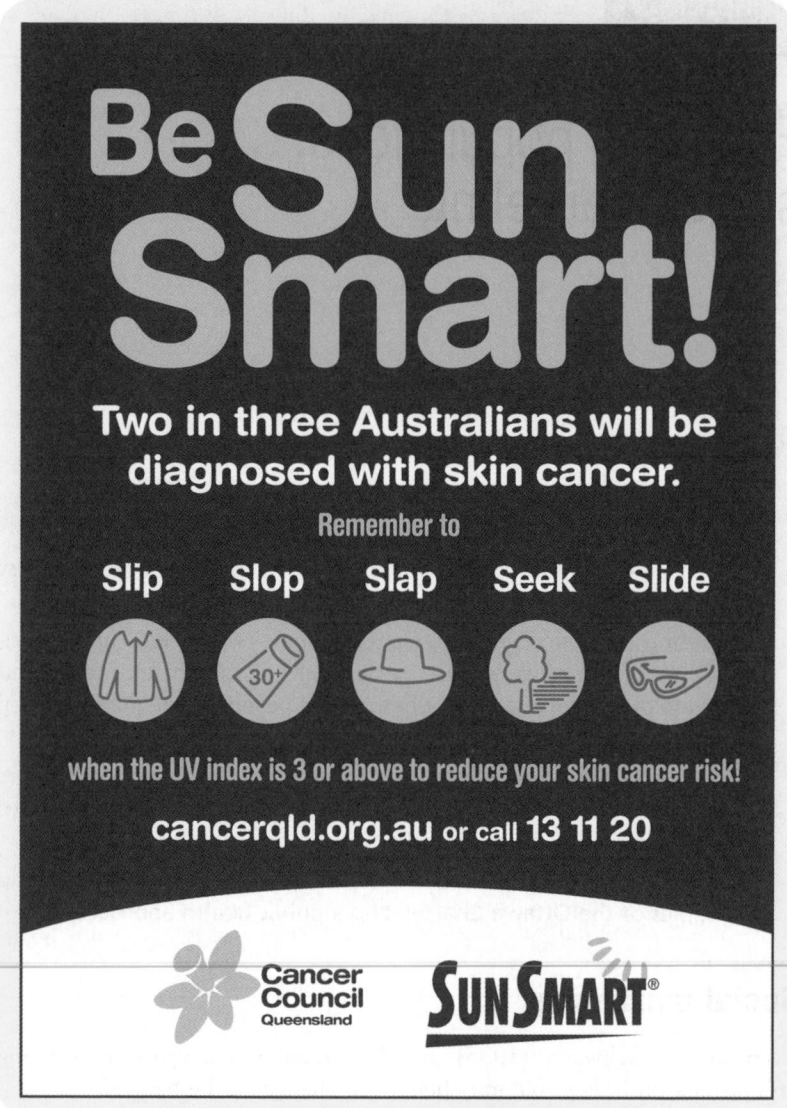

One of Australia's best known health slogans

Permission to reproduce the SunSmart logo and Slip Slop Slap Seek Slide slogan granted by Cancer Council Victoria

Australia and other industrialised nations as well as in developing countries. The 1980s saw massive growth, in Australia and overseas, of mass media-based health promotion campaigns utilising marketing tools, across a broad range of activities, including injury prevention, drinking and driving, seat belt usage, drugs, smoking, exercise, immunisation, nutrition and heart disease prevention (Egger, Donovan & Spark 1993; Fine 1990; Kotler & Roberto 1989; Manoff 1985; Walsh et al. 1993).

A number of factors influenced this trend. One was the realisation by social scientists and health professionals that, although they were expert in assessing what people should do, they were not necessarily expert in communicating these messages, or in motivating or facilitating behavioural change. Another influence was the apparent success of marketing techniques in the commercial area and the observation that the discipline of marketing provides a systematic, research-based approach for planning and implementing mass intervention programs.

Yet another influence was the move in public health towards the prevention of the so-called lifestyle diseases, such as heart disease and cancer—an approach based on epidemiological research findings about the relationships between habitual behaviours and long-term health outcomes. This focus on lifestyle diseases in turn led to an emphasis (some would say an undue emphasis) on individual responsibility and behaviour change. Hence, there was an increased acceptance of the marketing philosophy of individualism and rational free choice.

Some critics of social marketing have claimed that such a philosophy largely ignores the social, economic and environmental factors that influence individuals' health behaviour. Some social marketing campaigns deserve this criticism. However, it shows a lack of understanding of social marketing on both sides since one of the fundamental aspects of marketing—and hence social marketing—is an awareness of the total environment in which the organisation operates and how this environment influences, or can itself be influenced, to enhance the marketing activities of the company or health agency (see Donovan & Henley 2010; Hastings & Haywood 1994; Buchanan, Reddy & Hossain, 1994).

Social marketing defined

As first defined by Kotler and Zaltman (1971), social marketing is 'the design, implementation and control of programs calculated to influence the acceptability of social ideas and involving considerations of product planning, pricing, communications and market research'. A later and often-cited definition is that of Andreasen (1995): 'Social marketing is the application of commercial marketing technologies to the analysis, planning, execution, and evaluation of programs designed to influence the voluntary behaviour of target audiences in order to improve their personal welfare and that of their society'. These definitions indicate that 'social' marketing is just one 'branch' of marketing, where the branches reflect the area of application, for example, sports marketing, business-to-business or industrial marketing, not-for-profit marketing, events marketing, religious marketing and political marketing. However, the key point of difference to all other branches of marketing is that the social marketer's goal relates to the wellbeing of the community; for all others, the marketer's goal relates to the wellbeing of the marketer (e.g. sales and profits, members and donations, political representation). If the wellbeing of the community is not the goal, then it isn't social marketing (Donovan 2011).

Donovan and Henley (2010) consider Andreasen's definition too constrictive in its emphasis on voluntary behaviour. For example, they point out that a social marketing campaign for the Heart Foundation, which has an end goal of individuals consuming less saturated fat, might also target biscuit manufacturers to persuade them to substitute saturated fats in their products with polyunsaturated fats. While this requires a voluntary behaviour change among food company executives, the end-consumers' change in saturated fats intake is involuntary. Hence Donovan and Henley (2010) modify Andreasen's definition to: 'the application of commercial marketing technologies to the analysis, planning, execution and evaluation of programs designed to influence the voluntary or involuntary behaviour of target audiences in order to improve the welfare of individuals and society'. They also add two key points in their approach to social marketing:

- Given debate about who decides what is 'good' in the above definitions, they propose the United Nations Universal Declaration of Human Rights (www.un.org/en/documents/udhr) as the baseline with respect to the common good.
- Although most social marketing in the public health and injury prevention areas has focused on achieving individual behaviour change largely independent of the individual's social and economic circumstances, a primary future goal of social marketing is to achieve changes in the social determinants of health and wellbeing.

Under this approach, which is shared by other writers (e.g. Hastings, McFadyen & Anderson 2000; Andreasen 2006), social marketing is not just the targeting of individual voluntary behaviour change and changes to the environment that facilitate such changes but also the targeting of changes in social structures that will facilitate individuals reaching their potential. This includes targeting individuals in communities who have the power to make institutional policy and legislative change.

Social marketing uses key concepts from mainstream product and service marketing, such as: market segmentation; market research; competitive assessment; the use of product, price, promotion and distribution tactics; pre-testing and ongoing evaluation of campaign strategies; and models of consumer behaviour adapted from psychological and communications literature.

For many health promotion professionals, social marketing is seen as synonymous with the use of mass media to promote socially desirable causes.

This view is not unexpected, given that many social marketers see their basic product as information, or see social marketing as working primarily through channels of communication with information as its primary resource (Young 1989). However, in commercial marketing, the use of mass media is only one component of the total marketing process. For example, a product also must be designed to meet the buyer's 'needs'; it must be packaged and priced appropriately; it must be easily accessible; it should be 'trial-able' (if a large commitment is required); intermediaries such as wholesalers and retailers must be established; and, where relevant, sales staff must be informed and trained. Only after all these factors are in place is mass media used to make potential buyers:

- aware of the product
- aware of the product's benefits
- aware of where it can be purchased
- interested (i.e. motivated) to seek further information, or to purchase or trial the product.

In the same way, a campaign that aims to promote health by encouraging individual behaviour change must be based on more than just the mass media. Programs and strategies are required at the community level (i.e. they must be accessible); the activities promoted must be 'do-able' (i.e. within the target group's capacities) or learnable (i.e. skills must be defined and training must be available for specific activities); and they must be affordable. Social marketing, by definition, is a far more comprehensive and effective approach than simply using television advertising.

CASE STUDY **5.1**

Social marketing and drink-driving–related crashes

A systematic review of the effectiveness of mass media-supported campaigns for reducing alcohol-impaired driving (AID) and alcohol-related crashes was conducted in the US. In eight studies that met the criteria for inclusion in the review, the median decrease in alcohol-related crashes resulting from the campaigns was 13 per cent. Economic analyses of campaign effects indicated that the benefits to society were greater than the costs. The mass media-supported campaigns reviewed were generally carefully planned and well executed, attained adequate audience exposure, and were implemented in conjunction with other ongoing prevention activities, such as high-visibility enforcement. Hence there is strong evidence that, under these conditions, social marketing campaigns are effective in reducing AID and alcohol-related crashes.

Elder et al. 2004

117

Social marketing campaigns have been developed and implemented across a broad variety of areas, beginning largely in developing countries and dealing with issues such as rat control and other hygiene/sanitation issues, vaccination, family planning, agricultural methods and attitudes towards women (Manoff 1985). Applications in developed countries include a variety of areas, although the majority and most visible have been and continue to be in lifestyle factors related to health and injury prevention, including tobacco, HIV/AIDS, alcohol, drugs, nutrition and road safety, with lesser applications in other areas involving health and wellbeing, such as problem gambling, racism, child abuse and intimate partner violence, along with growing interest in applications to energy conservation, recycling and climate control (see Donovan and Henley 2010).

Social marketing in the health area (as practised by many health organisations) is marketing used to increase the effectiveness of public health and health promotion programs by providing principles and tools that more effectively reach and impact the target audiences for such programs. There are numerous examples from Australia and around the globe of public health campaigns benefiting from a marketing approach (see Cheng, Kotler & Lee 2010; French et al. 2010; Hornik 2002; Horsfall, Bromfield & McDonald 2010). Australia's road safety, sun protection and tobacco control programs are prime examples of incorporating marketing principles and tools to enhance success. These have all been substantially resourced, longstanding interventions.

In this chapter we first describe the fundamentals of traditional health promotion approaches that primarily target individuals to cease unhealthy behaviours and adopt healthy alternatives. We then propose a new social marketing that combines marketing fundamentals with the principles of the Ottawa Charter and the discipline of a public health approach to provide a framework for upstream interventions that target structural change.

Principles and practices of marketing

A number of aspects of consumer marketing have been discussed in the context of social marketing (Donovan & Henley 2010; Donovan & Owen 1994). Those most relevant for health promotion are: the marketing concept; the concept of exchange; customer value; market segmentation; competition and the principle of differential advantage; the use of market research; and the integration of the planning process. These concepts are discussed below.

1. The marketing concept: a consumer orientation

A customer focus is the essence of a marketing approach. Marketers seek profits or increased levels of participation in an activity or service through the identification of customer needs, the development of products and services to meet these needs, and the pricing, packaging, promotion and distribution of these products in accordance with consumer habits, aspirations and expectations.

A basic distinction between social and commercial marketing is that social marketing usually is not based on needs experienced by consumers but on needs identified by health experts. However, a marketing approach emphasises that the development, delivery and promotion of the health message and products or services must be carried out in accordance with consumers' needs. For example, messages about immunisation must be in a language consumers understand, the promised benefits must be relevant and the messages must be placed in media that consumers attend to.

2. The concept of exchange

The concept of exchange has long been described as the core concept of marketing: marketing is the exchange that takes place between consuming groups and supplying groups.

The essential factor that differentiates exchanges from other forms of need satisfaction is that each party to the exchange both gains and receives value. At the same time, each party perceives the offerings to involve costs. Hence it is the ratio of the perceived benefits to the costs that determines choice between alternatives (Kotler & Andreasen 1987). Kotler (1988) lists the following as necessary conditions for the potential for exchange:

1. There are at least two parties.
2. Each party offers something that might be of value to the other party.
3. Each party is capable of communication and delivery.
4. Each party is free to accept or reject the offer.
5. Each party believes it is appropriate or desirable to deal with the other party.

The lessons for social marketers are that we must offer something perceived to be of value to our target audiences and recognise that consumers must outlay resources, such as time, money, physical comfort, lifestyle changes or psychological effort, in exchange for the promised benefits. It also means that we must offer something of value to intermediaries, such as GPs, pharmacists and others whom we wish to involve in interventions.

3. Customer value: the concept of the marketing mix

There are two basic concepts with respect to customer value. First, customers do not just buy products or services, they buy benefits, or bundles of benefits.

Charles Revson of Revlon once said, 'In the factory we make cosmetics; in the store we sell hope.' Others have made the point that although someone might buy a quarter-inch drill (the product), what they want (the benefit) is a quarter-inch hole (Kotler 1988).

Second, the 'four Ps' of the marketing mix all contribute to customer value. The four Ps are:

- Product (e.g. brand name and reputation, packaging)
- Price (e.g. monetary cost, credit terms)

- Promotion (e.g. advertising, sales promotion, publicity and public relations, sponsorship, personal selling)
- Place or distribution (e.g. physical distribution, number and type of outlets, opening hours, atmosphere in outlets, availability of public transport, availability and ease of parking).

CASE STUDY **5.2**

Target marketing for health checks

As part of a project to encourage men to visit their doctor for a check-up, Cancer Council Western Australia placed the ad below in the sporting news section of the daily newspaper. The ad occupied half a page and had a 'male interest' headline to attract attention. The advertisement included a self-assessment questionnaire to attract readers to the content of the ad and, it was hoped, to trigger some action if the score indicated that action was required. This approach was based on research that suggested that men like to have health feedback in the nature of 'a score'. A telephone number was included to provide further information to those who called.

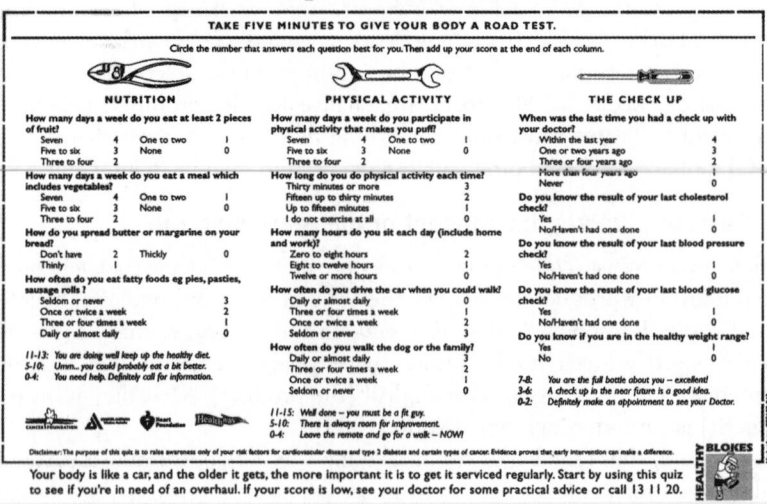

Cancer Council Western Australia

The marketing manager's task is to blend these four elements to provide maximal value to particular market segments. For example, time and effort costs are reduced by making the product easily obtainable (e.g. wide distribution, vending machines in appropriate locations, online ordering); 'trial-able' before commitment (e.g. sample packs, in-office/in-home demonstrations, 'seven-day free trial'); easy to pay for (e.g. credit card acceptance, lay-by, hire purchase); and easy to use (e.g. user-friendly packaging, instructions on use, free training courses).

A concept that ties these two aspects (customer benefits and the four Ps) together is Kotler's (1988) concept of the core product, the augmented product and the actual, tangible product. For example, the tangible product might be a computer; the augmented product involves after-sales service, training, warranties, associated software, a widespread consumer user network, and so on; the core product is better management decision making. Many companies primarily compete not on tangible product features but on augmented product features (Levitt 1969).

In the health promotion of physical activity, the core product might be a longer, healthier life by means of cardiovascular disease risk reduction, the actual product might be an aerobics class, and the augmented product might include a crèche, off-peak discount rates, clean, hygienic change rooms and a complimentary towel.

A fifth P—People—applies to services, something particularly appropriate in health promotion. Domestic violence helpline counsellors, for example, need extensive and appropriate training to deal with violent callers and encourage them to join perpetrator programs (Donovan, Paterson, Francas 1999; Donovan et al. 2000; see Case study 5.3).

4. Market segmentation: the principle of selectivity and concentration

Market segmentation involves dividing the total market into groups of individuals that are more like each other than like individuals in other groups. The fundamental issue is to identify groups that will respond differently to different products or marketing strategies, and, for commercial organisations, to select and concentrate on those segments for which the organisation can be most competitive.

The segmentation process has three phases:

1. dividing the total market into segments and developing profiles of these segments
2. evaluating each segment and selecting one or more segments as target markets
3. developing a detailed marketing mix (i.e. the 4Ps) for each of the selected segments.

CASE STUDY **5.3**

The Freedom from Fear campaign marketing mix

The Western Australian Freedom from Fear campaign encouraged violent and potentially violent men to call a men's domestic violence helpline, where counsellors would then attempt to persuade the callers to enrol in counselling programs. The primary medium for reaching violent and potentially violent men was television advertising (especially in sporting programs), supported by radio advertising and posters. Extensive formative research was undertaken to ensure acceptance of the advertisement messages by the target group without negatively affecting victims, children and relevant stakeholders.

The helpline was staffed by counsellors (people specifically trained to deal with violent men), who were able to assess callers and conduct lengthy telephone counselling (i.e. product) with members of the target audience. Anonymity was assured, and there was no pressure on the men. The primary aim of the helpline counsellors was to refer as many callers as possible into no-fee (i.e. price) government-funded counselling programs provided primarily by private sector organisations in 12 locations throughout the state (i.e. place). This pricing strategy was necessary to ensure that victims of low-income perpetrators would not be disadvantaged by their partner's limited income. Programs were time scheduled (i.e. place) to allow employed men access to programs in non-working hours (i.e. consumer orientation).

The core product—that is, the end benefit being offered to violent men in relationships in exchange for their acceptance of counselling—was the opportunity to keep their relationship (or family) intact by ending the violence towards their partner (and its effect on children). Other products included self-help booklets providing tips on how to control violence and how to contact service providers. These were also provided on audio-cassettes for men with poor reading skills (i.e. consumer orientation).

Donovan & Henley 2003

The concept of market segmentation is fundamental to developing communication campaigns and is dealt with in detail below.

Segmentation for health promotion

One of the basic distinctions between health promotion campaigns and commercial marketing campaigns is that health promotion campaigns are usually based not on needs experienced by consumers but on needs identified by health experts or government health authorities (Sirgy, Morris & Samli 1985). This often leads to a lack of segmentation of an audience and hence a scattergun approach to delivering a message. A focus on consumer or client needs naturally calls for a segmentation of the prospective audience since it is obvious that vastly different sub-groups exist in a population, that the differences occur in a variety of dimensions (or bases), and that different strategies and approaches are necessary to reach and communicate effectively with these different sub-groups.

CASE STUDY **5.4**

Example advertisement: Targeting by risk factor status

Skin cancer
Have you been checked?
The ..... LIONS CLUB has organised a FREE skin cancer screening. Specialists from the LIONS CANCER INSTITUTE will be available to examine people who feel they are at risk of having skin cancer.

If you are 16 years of age or older and have one or more of the following:

- a family member who has had a malignant melanoma
- five or more moles (not freckles) on your arms
- previously had moles or skin cancer removed
- a mole or freckle that is changing size or colour
- fair skin that burns rather than tans
- had blistering sunburn as a child
- any inflamed skin sores that do not heal

   then please phone .... to make an appointment.
   Venue: ....
   Date: ....
If you are concerned but cannot attend the screening on that date, please express your interest with the LIONS CANCER INSTITUTE and see your family doctor.

For health promotion campaigns, target groups are often described in terms of risk factors (e.g. smokers, the obese, the inactive, heavy drinkers, diabetics) or demographic groupings that epidemiologically appear to be at higher risk (e.g. blue-collar groups, sedentary occupations, remote Aboriginal communities, street kids). Regardless of the base(s) chosen for the initial segmentation (e.g. age and gender), the segments are also usually described or profiled on as many other variables as possible, so as to better understand the chosen segment(s). However, we consider that two fundamental segmentation approaches are useful in social marketing health campaigns: stage segmentation and attitude–behaviour segmentation. These are useful segmentations because the campaign strategies follow directly from the underlying segmentation models.

123

As described in Chapter 2, Prochaska and colleagues (1994) divides the total target segment (e.g. smokers) into sub-segments depending on their stage in progression towards adoption of a desired type of behaviour (i.e. quitting smoking):

1. *Precontemplation*—where the individual is not even considering modifying their unhealthy behaviour.
2. *Contemplation*—where the individual is considering changing their unhealthy behaviour, but not in the immediate future.
3. *Preparation*—where the individual plans to try to change their unhealthy behaviour in the immediate future (i.e. in the next 2 weeks or an appropriate time frame).
4. *Action*—the immediate (6-month) period following trial and adoption of the recommended behaviour and cessation of the unhealthy behaviour.
5. *Maintenance*—the period following the action stage until the unhealthy behaviour is fully extinguished.
6. *Termination*—when the problem behaviour is completely eliminated; that is, zero temptation across all problem situations.

Donovan and Owen (1994) claim that health promotion campaigns relying mainly on mass media are most influential in the precontemplation and contemplation stages (by raising the salience and personal relevance of the issue), of moderate influence in the preparation stage (by reinforcing perceptions of self-efficacy and maintaining salience of the perceived benefits of adopting the recommended behaviour), and of least influence in the action and maintenance stages, where beliefs and attitudes are well established and where socio-environmental influences on the achieved behaviour are greatest. A number of studies have shown that different message and intervention strategies are more or less appropriate for people in the different stages (Prochaska et al. 1994).

Attitude–behaviour segmentation: the Sheth–Frazier model

Sheth and Frazier (1982) developed a model of strategy mix choice for behaviour change. They suggest that there are four major processes of planned social change, each one most appropriate for each of four combinations of attitude–behaviour consistency or discrepancy (see Table 5.1).

Survey data provide the proportion of the population of interest in each of these cells, with the cell designation indicating the appropriate strategy for each cell. That is, when attitudes and behaviour are consistent and in the desired direction with respect to the relevant behaviour (cell 1), a reinforcement process is called for to sustain the desired behaviour. This can be done by (a) reinforcing the attitude, (b) reinforcing the behaviour, or both. For example, people who are both predisposed towards exercise and carry out regular exercise can be encouraged to continue to do so by reminding them of the benefits of exercise or by making it easier to carry

Table 5.1: A typology of strategy mix for planned social change

| | ATTITUDE | |
	Positive	Negative
	Cell 1	Cell 2
Perform	Reinforcement process	Rationalisation process
		Attitude change
DESIRED BEHAVIOUR		
	Cell 3	Cell 4
Don't perform	Inducement process	Confrontation process
	Behaviour change	

Sheth & Frazier 1982

out their exercise routine. If attitudes are positive but the behaviour is not being performed (cell 3), an inducement process aimed at minimising or removing organisational, socioeconomic, time and place constraints (such as improving availability of exercise facilities) should be used.

Where the behaviour is being performed but the attitude is negative (cell 2), rationalisation is most appropriate (e.g. relating exercise to good health). Where attitudes are negative and the behaviour is not being performed (cell 4), a confrontational approach might be necessary (e.g. a face-to-face warning by a GP to an individual of the health risks of not taking any exercise).

5. Competition and the principle of differential advantage

In marketing, competition and differential advantage refer to an analysis of the marketer's resources versus those of the competition, with the aim of determining where the company enjoys a differential advantage over the opposition. In a wider sense it relates to monitoring and understanding competitive activity, sometimes to emulate or follow such activity, in other cases to pre-empt or counter competitors' activities.

In health promotion, it is necessary to identify, understand and develop counter strategies for the competition. A study of alcohol advertising and promotion, for example, can assist in understanding appeals to young people (Jones & Donovan 2001) and for identifying breaches of the Alcohol Beverages Advertising Code (Jones & Donovan 2002; Donovan, Fielder & Jalleh 2011). Similarly, advocacy groups need to monitor such industries as the tobacco and food industries and attempt to pre-empt industry marketing tactics that have a negative influence on children and other vulnerable groups. For example, many non-nutritious snack foods offer convenience, low price, good taste and a fun image. To compete, healthy snack foods must satisfy these same needs, or introduce 'new' benefits that are attractive to people.

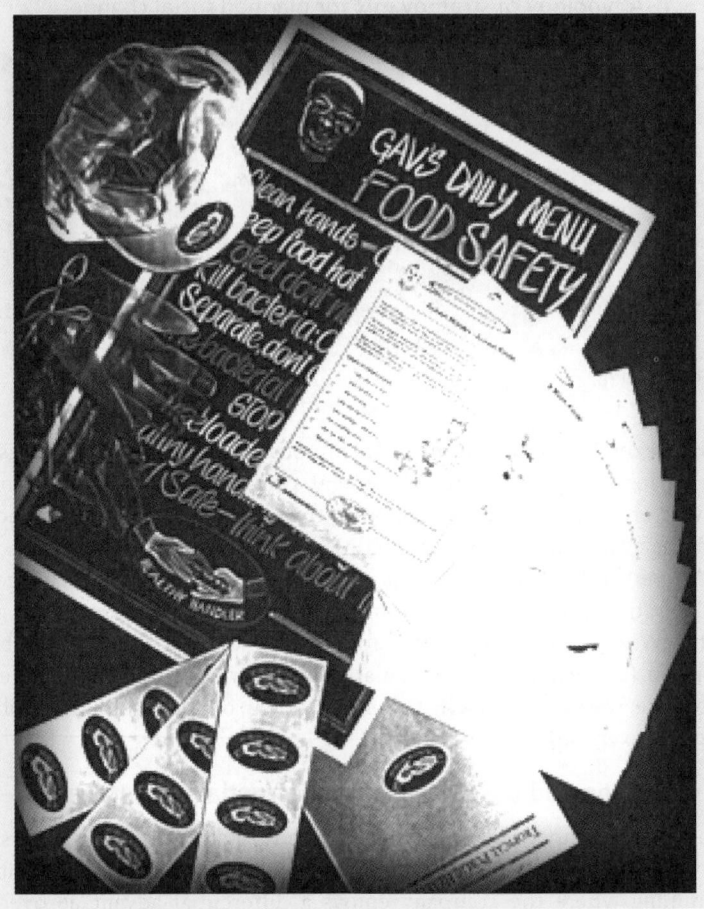

Materials promoting good hygiene for food handlers in North Queensland as part of Queensland Health's Foodsafe campaign

Categorising the competition

Donovan and Henley (2010) propose the following categories to assist in designing strategies to monitor and counter the competition:

- competitors clearly defined by the fact that any use of their products could be harmful (e.g. tobacco, some illicit drugs, leaded petrol, some forms of asbestos)
- competitors defined by the fact that excess use or abuse of their products is harmful (e.g. foods high in salt, sugar and saturated fats; illicit drugs; alcohol; guns; motor vehicles; gambling; videogames and movies containing sex and violence)

- competitors defined by beliefs and values that inhibit the uptake of healthy behaviours (e.g. attitudes to birth control inhibiting family planning; machismo attitudes inhibiting condom use and facilitating the spread of AIDS; attitudes to women that condone violence against women; attitudes and values that affect the health of the planet in general, such as materialism; consumption as lifestyle)
- competitors defined by beliefs and values that create conflict in society (e.g. racist organisations; fundamentalist religious organisations; terrorist groups)
- competitors defined by beliefs and values that may have negative consequences for many, while benefiting a select few (e.g. global corporations; privatisation of government services; armaments suppliers; global media organisations).

6. The use of market research

Given all of the above, it should be apparent that effective marketing is a research-based process. Research in social marketing is concerned both with epidemiological data and with assessment of such factors as: what health 'products' (e.g. exercise, dietary fat reduction, smoking cessation) the community perceives as priorities for action; what tangible products can be developed to facilitate the adoption of health-promoting behaviour or to reduce risk (e.g. no-tar cigarettes, low-fat foods, quit smoking kits, exercise videos); what programs or services can be offered (e.g. weight control, aerobics classes, educational videos on the benefits of exercise; training videos on how to institute worksite programs); how the message strategy should be developed; what social and structural facilitators and inhibitors need to be taken into account; who the relevant influencers and intermediaries are; which media (television, radio, press, internet) and which media vehicles (specific programs), if any, can be used to reach the target audience(s) cost-effectively; and what activities are being undertaken by 'anti-health' marketers.

7. An integrated planning process

The marketing process is an integrated process such that elements of the marketing mix, the organisation's resources, the use of market research, and the selection and concentration on specific market segments are all combined to maximise the value of the organisation's offerings to the consumer, and hence profit to the company. For health organisations, this integration is intended to maximise intended changes in knowledge, attitude or behaviour among individuals in the community, planners, policy makers and public servants.

This integration strongly implies the need for a systematic strategic planning process: the setting of clearly defined overall goals; the setting of measurable objectives to meet the overall goals; the delineation of strategies and tactics to achieve these objectives; and management and feedback systems to ensure that the plan is implemented as desired and to avert or deal with problems as they arise.

Differences between commercial and social marketing: can we sell health like we sell soap?

Although the principles and practices of marketing are clearly applicable to the promotion of healthy lifestyles, it is a mistake to assume that social marketing is similar to commercial marketing in all respects. Even within marketing, different approaches are more or less appropriate for different products. In short, although some of the principles of marketing are applicable, selling health or any other socially desirable product cannot be fully equated with selling soap.

Bloom and Novelli (1981) and Rothschild (1979) list a number of important differences between the marketing of commercial products and social marketing. The major differences are:

1. Commercial products tend to offer instant gratification whereas the benefits of healthy behaviour are often delayed.
2. Social marketing attempts to replace undesirable behaviour with behaviour that is often more costly in time or effort and, at least in the short term, less pleasurable or in fact unpleasant.
3. Commercial marketing mostly aims at groups already positive towards the product and its benefits, whereas social marketing often is directed towards hard-to-reach, at-risk groups who are often most antagonistic to change.
4. Health risk behaviours are often extremely complex, both at a personal and at a social level, and far more so than behaviours involved in purchasing and consuming most commercial products.
5. Intermediaries in commercial marketing are far fewer in type and generally far easier to deal with (although perhaps more costly) than in social marketing.
6. Defining and communicating the product is far more difficult in social marketing, especially where different experts might have different views on the subject.
7. The exchange process is far easier to define in commercial marketing than in social marketing.
8. Much targeted health-related behaviour is inconsistent with social pressures.
9. Ethical questions and issues of equity are far more complex and important (e.g. victim blaming) in social marketing.
10. Social marketing should be directed towards not just changes in individual behaviour but also to changes in systems and social structures that operate to the detriment of the health of populations.

The techniques and principles of marketing are applicable to any consumer decision, yet their effective application to health promotion requires an understanding of both areas. In practical terms this requires close cooperation between marketing experts, public health professionals, and, for mass media campaign components, behavioural scientists with expertise in communication theory and attitude and behaviour change.

Going upstream—social marketing's 'new 4Ps'

Social marketing for health combines the principles of marketing, the principles of the Ottawa Charter and the principles of a public health approach (Figure 5.1). Back in 1986, the Ottawa Charter explicitly stated that health promotion should not only target individual undesirable behaviours but also act to create social, political, health-service and legislative environments that support communities and individuals to make desirable changes. However, almost all early health promotion campaigns—and even many recent ones—largely targeted individual risk behaviours with little attention to the environments in which health promotion takes place (e.g. schools, workplaces, cities). Although the emphasis remains on the individual in some campaigns (such as the Australian Government's Measure Up campaign), many health promotion programs are including these 'upstream' objectives in their programs, particularly as the health

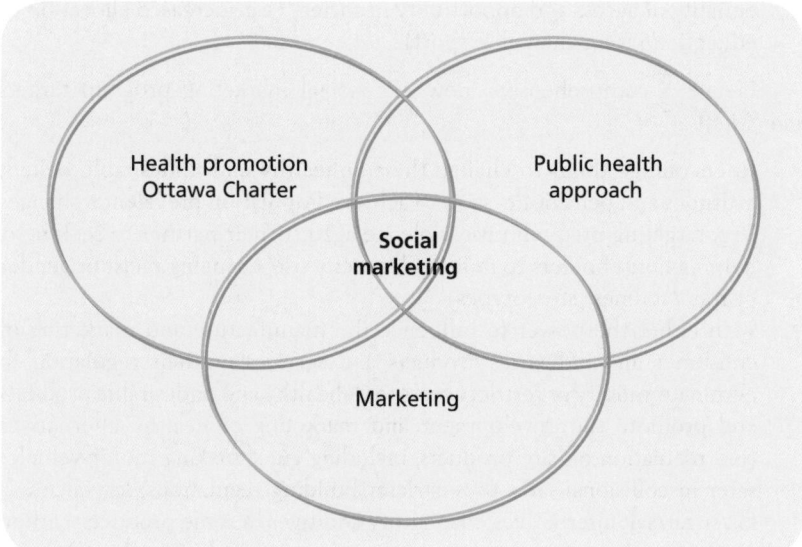

Figure 5.1: Social marketing for health

129

promotion approach is being increasingly accepted as more effective than the traditional health education approach by public health professionals who bring a broader, upstream perspective to such programs. Marketing principles also can be used to help focus on these upstream objectives.

In addition to commercial marketing's basic 4Ps (Price, Place, Promotion, Product), applying marketing to the concepts of health promotion and public health suggests new, additional 4Ps for social marketing. These new, additional '4Ps' represent the goals of social marketing in the context of health promotion's Ottawa Charter, the public health approach and the need for change at a societal political level (see Maibach, Abroms & Marosits 2007 and Cohen, Scribner & Farley 2000 for similar but more limited frameworks). These 4Ps emphasise the need to modify environmental influences on behaviour along with upstream social determinants factors (Donovan 2011). These 4P goals are to achieve changes in the:

- Population prevalence of individual undesirable, unhealthy or risky behaviours (e.g. smoking rates, physical activity, incidence of child abuse)
- design and/or marketing of Products people use or consume that impact on health and wellbeing (e.g. healthier food products, restrictions on alcohol marketing, pre-set limits on gambling machines)
- design and/or marketing of Places where people live, work and play so as to reduce harm and enhance wellbeing (e.g. safer children's playgrounds, automatic teller machines banned from gambling venues)
- Political structure that allocates resources so as to ensure increased equality of access and opportunity in society (e.g. increased allocation to education rather than elite sport).

Hence, a comprehensive 'new 4Ps' social marketing program targets *individuals:*

- to encourage them to change their unhealthy and undesirable beliefs, attitudes and behaviours so as to achieve Population prevalence changes (e.g. targeting men who use violence against their partner to seek help, helping householders to reduce electricity use, changing racist or gender or mental illness stereotypes)
- with either the power to influence the manufacture and marketing of consumer and industrial Products and services or their regulation to eliminate, modify or restrict access to unhealthy and undesirable products and promote the development and marketing of healthy alternatives (e.g. regulation of 'sin' products, including guns; making motor vehicles safer in collisions; safer toys; stricter building regulations; low-alcohol/fat/sugar/salt alternatives; mandatory additives in some products; carbon emission reduction technology; slower operating poker machines)
- with the power to make changes to and regulate activities in Places where people congregate (e.g. worksites, schools, recreational areas, institutions/

hospitals, sporting venues) to facilitate healthy, positive behaviours and reduce risky behaviours (e.g. safe exercise areas, safe serving practices in bars, regulations to prevent overcrowding, shade sails over swimming pools, reduction of lead emissions, safe rail crossings, canteens with healthy foods, no-smoking areas, urban design to reduce crime)

* who have Political power to determine the allocation of a society's financial and other resources and to change public institutions such as the media and the law, and government bureaucracies such as education and health services, to ensure equality of access and opportunity as per the Universal Declaration of Human Rights.

It is in this last area that public health professionals and social marketers need to cooperate with and learn lessons from social medicine, liberation theology, civil rights movements, legal activists and others (see Ackerman & DuVall 2001).

Overall, coupling the traditional marketing framework with the new 4Ps framework is more likely to result in a comprehensive program, and hence a greater likelihood of sustained effectiveness. This applies not only to the health area, but to all areas of application where the objective is the social good.

CASE STUDY **5.5**

Community-based social marketing to promote positive mental health: the Act–Belong–Commit campaign (actbelongcommit.org.au)

Developed by a team based at Curtin University in Western Australia, the Act–Belong–Commit campaign is a population-based mental health promotion campaign. The campaign combines a community development and social marketing approach to improve community understanding of positive mental health and to involve health and non-health related service providers in promoting good mental health.

The campaign targets individuals to engage in activities that enhance their mental health while encouraging campaign and community partners (e.g. health service providers, local government organisations, and community sports, arts and service organisations that provide mentally healthy activities) to promote their activities under the banner of the Act–Belong–Commit message (Donovan, James & Jalleh 2007; Jalleh et al. 2007). Specifically, the campaign's messages are that keeping mentally, physically and socially active (*Act*), participating in group-based activities by joining formal and informal community groups (*Belong*), and having meaning and purpose in life by taking up realistic challenges, setting goals and getting involved in a cause or volunteering (*Commit*) are the foundations of good mental health. There is considerable scientific evidence that these three domains of behaviour contribute to good mental health (see Donovan, James et al. 2006).

The execution of this evidence-based campaign was developed primarily from research into people's perceptions of mental health and the behaviours they believed protected and promoted good mental health (Donovan et al. 2003; Donovan, Henley et al. 2006)

131

Feeling Blue? Act Green!

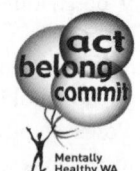

Mentally Healthy WA

It seems that watching wildlife shows, exploring parks and gardens, looking at fabulous mountain and ocean views, and getting away from it all to the bush and Pacific island beaches are not only pleasurable, but are actually good for us!

Eminent biologists, psychologists and health professionals are showing that contact with nature — whether through parks, natural bush, pets or farm animals — helps us recover from stress and mental fatigue, helps us relax and puts us in a good frame of mind.

Of course, most of us know this intuitively and it's probably why we are drawn to nature instinctively. We all know that a walk on the beach, down a bush track or in a park is good to clear the head when we feel a little tired or stressed.

So, next time you are feeling like a lift, 'act green': do some gardening, pet the cat or dog, take a walk around the park or head down to the water for some time out.

Better still, don't wait until you're tired or feeling flat. Act green more often. Being in touch with nature makes us feel good, builds good mental health and helps beat the blues. And it's as easy as A-B-C!

Act: do some gardening; take a walk around the local park; watch a wildlife documentary; take time to watch the sun set; spend time with pets...

Belong: get a group together for a picnic in a natural setting; visit a wildlife sanctuary with friends; join a hiking group...

Commit: become a 'civic environmentalist'; join a tree planting group; volunteer to keep your local parks & gardens clean; take up orienteering; learn more about ecology; offer to take a home-bound person out to a park...

Being active, having a sense of belonging, and having a purpose in life all contribute to happiness and good mental health.

(08) 9266 3788
actbelongcommit.org.au

A poster for the Act-Belong-Commit campaign

Courtesy of the Act-Belong-Commit campaign coordinated by Mentally Healthy WA

Concluding comments

Social marketing can be viewed at one level as simply a bag of tools or technologies adapted from commercial marketing and applied to issues for the social good. A key point is the marketing concept or 'philosophy' that emphasises the perspective of the target audience as the basis for achieving mutually satisfying exchanges. From a broader perspective, social marketing in the health area is the application of commercial marketing techniques in the context of the Ottawa Charter and the public health paradigm, so as to achieve individual behaviour changes and societal structural changes consistent with the United Nations Universal Declaration of Human Rights. However, the US National Academy of Sciences' Institute of Medicine (2000) report into social and behavioural intervention strategies for health concluded that although environment-based strategies have the greatest population effect, far more progress had been made in developing individual-oriented interventions than environmental-oriented interventions. The new 4Ps are a way to help redress this situation. It is noted that Australia's National Preventative Health Taskforce has recommended that social marketing strategies be adopted for the three main areas identified for action in Australia (obesity, alcohol, tobacco). The new 4Ps are consistent with various aspects of the taskforce's recommendations, including the emphasis on engaging communities (changes in places) and influencing markets (changes in products and their regulation). The taskforce also noted the need to reduce inequalities that influenced the three main action areas. To achieve this turnaround (changes in political priorities), future applications of social marketing will need to work alongside practitioners in, and incorporate lessons and principles from, areas such as social medicine, social activism, social entrepreneurship and civic engagement.

References

Ackerman, P., & DuVall, J., 2001, *A Force More Powerful*, Palgrave/St Martin's Press, New York.

Andreasen, A.R., 1995, *Marketing Social Change: Changing Behaviour to Promote Health, Social Development, and the Environment*, Jossey-Bass, San Francisco.

Andreasen, A.R., 2006, *Social Marketing in the 21st Century*, Sage, California.

Bloom, P.N., & Novelli, W.D., 1981, Problems and challenges of social marketing, *J Marketing* 45:79–88.

Buchanan, D.R., Reddy, S., & Hossain, Z., 1994, Social marketing: a critical appraisal, *Health Promot Int* 9:49–57.

Cheng, H., Kotler, P., & Lee, N.R., 2010, *Social Marketing in Public Health: Global Trends and Success Stories*, Jones and Bartlett Publishers, Sudbury, Massachusetts.

Cohen, D., Scribner, R., & Farley, T., 2000, A structural model of health behavior: a pragmatic approach to explain and influence health behaviors at the population level, *Prev Med* 30(2):146–54.

Donovan, R.J., 2011, Social marketing's mythunderstandings, *J Soc Marketing* 1(1):8–16.

Donovan, R.J., Fielder, L., & Jalleh, G., 2011, Alcohol advertising advocacy research no match for corporate dollars: the case of Bundy R Bear, *J Res Consumers* 20.

Donovan, R.J., Francas, M., Paterson, D., & Zappelli, R., 2000, Formative research for mass media-based campaigns: Western Australia's 'Freedom from Fear' campaign targeting male perpetrators of intimate partner violence, *Health Promot J Aust* 10(2):78–83.

Donovan, R.J., & Henley, N., 2003, *Social Marketing: Principles and Practice*, IP Communications, Melbourne.

Donovan, R.J., & Henley, N., 2010, *Social Marketing: An International Perspective*, Cambridge University Press, Cambridge.

Donovan, R.J., Henley, N., Jalleh, G., Silburn, S., Zubrick, S., & Williams, A., 2006, The impact on mental health in others of those in a position of authority: a perspective of parents, teachers, trainers and supervisors, *Aust eJournal Advancement Mental Health* [online] 5(1):60–6, available at www.auseinet.com/journal/vol5iss1/donovan.pdf.

Donovan, R.J., James, R., & Jalleh, G., 2007, Community-based social marketing to promote positive mental health: the Act-Belong-Commit campaign in rural Western Australia, in Hastings, G. (Ed.) *Social Marketing: Why Should the Devil Have All the Best Tunes?*, Butterworth Heinemann, London.

Donovan, R.J., James, R., Jalleh, G., & Sidebottom, C., 2006, Implementing mental health promotion: the Act–Belong–Commit Mentally Healthy WA campaign in Western Australia, *Int J Mental Health Promot* 8(1):33–42.

Donovan, R.J., & Owen, N., 1994, Social marketing and population interventions, in Dishman, R.K. (Ed.), *Advances in Exercise Adherence* (2nd edn), Human Kinetics Publishers, Champaign, Illinois.

Donovan, R.J., Paterson, D., & Francas, M., 1999, Targeting male perpetrators of intimate partner violence: Western Australia's 'Freedom from Fear' campaign, *Soc Marketing Quarterly* 5(3):127–43.

Donovan, R.J., Watson, N., Henley, N., Williams, A., Silburn, S., Zubrick, S., James, R., Cross, D., Hamilton, G., & Roberts, C., 2003, *Mental Health Promotion Scoping Project, Report to Healthway*, Centre for Behavioural Research in Cancer Control, Curtin University, Western Australia.

Egger, G., Donovan, R.J., & Spark, R., 1993, *Health and the Media: Principles and Practice for Health Promotion*, McGraw-Hill, Sydney.

Elder, R.W., Shults, R.A., Sleet, D.A., Nichols, J.L., Thompson, R.S., & Rajab, W., 2004, Effectiveness of mass media campaigns for reducing drinking and driving and alcohol-involved crashes: a systematic review, *Am J Prev Med* 27(1):57–65.

Fine, S.H., 1990, *The Marketing of Ideas and Social Issues* (2nd edn), Praeger, New York.

French, J., Blair-Stevens, C., McVey, D., & Merritt, R., 2010, *Social Marketing and Public Health: Theory and Practice*, Oxford University Press, Oxford.

Hastings, G., & Haywood, A., 1994, Social marketing: a critical response, *Health Promot Int* 9:59–63.

Hastings, G., McFadyen, L., & Anderson, S., 2000, Whose behaviour is it anyway? The broader potential of social marketing, *Soc Marketing Quarterly* 6(2):46–58.

Hornik, R.C. (Eed.), 2002, *Public Health Communication: Evidence for Behaviour Change*, Lawrence Erlbaum Associates, New Jersey.

Horsfall, B., Bromfield, L., & McDonald, M., 2010, Are social marketing campaigns effective in preventing child abuse and neglect?, *NCPC Issues:* 32:1–28.

Jalleh, G., Donovan, R.J., James, R., & Ambridge, J., 2007, Process evaluation of the Act–Belong–Commit Mentally Health WA campaign: first 12 months data, *Health Promot J Aust* 18(3):217–20.

Jones, S., & Donovan, R.J., 2001, Messages in alcohol advertising targeted to youth, *Aust N Z J Public Health* 25(2):126–31.

Jones, S., & Donovan, R.J., 2002, Self-regulation of alcohol advertising: is it working for Australia?, *J Public Affairs* 2(3):153–65.

Kotler, P., 1988, *Marketing Management: Analysis, Planning, Implementation and Control*, Prentice Hall, Englewood Cliffs, NJ.

Kotler, P., & Andreasen, A.R., 1987, *Strategic Marketing for Nonprofit Organisations*, Prentice Hall, Englewood Cliffs, NJ.

Kotler, P., & Roberto, E.L., 1989, *Social Marketing: Strategies for Changing Public Behaviour*, Free Press, New York.

Kotler, P., & Zaltman, G., 1971, Social marketing: an approach to planned social change, *J Marketing* 35:3–12.

Levitt, T., 1969, *The Marketing Mode*, McGraw-Hill, New York.

Maibach, E., Abroms, L., & Marosits, M., 2007, Communication and marketing as tools to cultivate the public's health: a proposed 'people and places' framework, *BMC Public Health*, 7(88), doi:10.1186/1471-2458-7-88.

Manoff, R.K., 1985, *Social Marketing*, Praeger, New York.

National Academy of Sciences, Institute of Health (US), 2000, *Promoting Health: Intervention Strategies from Social and Behavioral Research*, National Academies Press, Washington, DC.

Prochaska, J.O., Velicer, W.F., Rossi, J.S., Goldstein, M.G., Marcus, B.H., Rakowski, W., Fiore, C., Harlow, L.L., Redding, C.A., Rosenbloom, D., & Rossi, S.R., 1994, Stages of change and decisional balance for 12 problem behaviours, *Health Psychol* 13:39–46.

Rothschild, M.L., 1979, Marketing communications in non-business situations or why it's so hard to sell brotherhood like soap, *J Marketing* 43:11–20.

Schwartz, B., 1995, *Social Marketing Workshop*, Academy for Educational Development, Washington, DC.

Sheth, J.N., & Frazier, G.L., 1982, A model of strategy mix choice for planned social change, *J Marketing* 46:15–26.

Sirgy, M.J., Morris, M., & Samli, A.C., 1985, The question of value in social marketing: use of a quality-of-life theory to achieve long-term satisfaction, *Am J Econ Sociol* 44:215–28.

Walsh, D.C., Rudd, R.E., Moeykens, B.A., & Moloney, T.W., 1993, Social marketing for public health, *Health Affairs* 12:104–19.

Young, E., 1989, Social marketing in the information era, Paper presented to the American Marketing Association Conference, Social Marketing for the 1990s, Ottawa.

chapter 6

Focus on populations: the media

Summary of main points

- The media—in all forms—is a crucial component of social marketing and health promotion campaigns, given that our major 'product' is often information.

- There are five major media methods: advertising, publicity, edutainment, civic journalism and word of mouth (including through social media).

- There are three major media campaign objectives: informing, persuading and advocating.

- Choice of method and delivery channel depends on campaign objectives, target audiences and available resources.

Using the media

The availability and types of media channels today have expanded substantially since the first edition of this book in 1990. However, while the newer channels (e.g. internet, mobile phones, electronic tablets) are undoubtedly important, Donovan and Henley (2010) note that recent global award-winning advertising campaigns have been characterised by an emphasis on what people are now calling 'traditional' media channels: commercial television, commercial radio, print and out-of-home media (Dawson 2009; Lannon 2008). We take the view that it is not the media channels per se that are of interest, but how they are used to achieve one's objectives. In our view, innovative use of media does not equate only to technology; rather it equates to identifying locations (or 'touchpoints') where we can reach, engage and impact our target audiences (Manning 2009) and to strategic use of creative executions that generate publicity and action. That is, we need to be creative in reaching target audience members at critical times. Hence the placement of anti-drug advertising in bathrooms at bars and nightclubs, 'Keep It Safe. Keep It Hidden. Keep It Locked' signs at parking areas, roadside road safety billboards, drive-time road safety ads on radio, sun-protection warnings at beaches and swimming pools, and messages delivered by mobile phone at appropriate times.

In this chapter we will cover the main methods of using the media (advertising; publicity; edutainment; civic journalism; word-of-mouth, including through social media) and the major objectives for media campaigns regardless of the channel used. We will mention, but not discuss in depth, the main channels available and how the newer channels are being used in social marketing and health promotion, given that the newer technologies will no doubt change rapidly over the next few years. See Table 6.1 for a summary of the most frequently used media vehicles.

Table 6.1:   A summary of main media vehicles and their characteristics

Type: Limited reach	Characteristics
Pamphlets/brochures	Information transmission. Best where cognition, rather than emotion, is desired outcome. Downloadable.
Fact/information sheets	Quick, convenient information. Use as series with storage folder. Not for complex behaviour change. Downloadable.
Newsletters	Continuity. Personalised. Labour-intensive and requires detailed commitment and needs assessment before commencing. Easily widely distributed by email.
Posters	Agenda-setting function. Visual message. Creative input required. Possibility of graffiti might be considered.
T-shirts	Emotive. Personal. Useful for cementing attitudes and commitment to program/idea.
Stickers	Short messages to identify/motivate the user and cement commitment. Cheap, persuasive.
Wallet cards	Much like stickers. Useful for reminder information and helpline numbers.
Videos	Instructional. Motivational. Useful for personal viewing with adults as back-up to other programs.
DVDs and CDs	Provide the opportunity for portable, attractive easy to use, multimedia transmitted information.
Cinema	Captive audience. Can target to specific audiences. Emotive potential given large screen.
Podcasts	Digital audio, video, pdf files downloadable by subscription.

continued

Table 6.1: *continued*

Mass reach	Characteristics
Television	Awareness, arousal, modelling and image creation role. May be increasingly useful in information and skills training as awareness and interest in health increases. Mainstreaming readily available.
Radio	Informative, interactive (talkback). Cost-effective and useful in creating awareness, providing information.
Newspapers	Print and digital. Long and short copy information. Material dependent on type of newspaper and day of week.
Magazines	Print and digital. Wide readership and influence. Useful in supportive role and to inform and provide social proof.
Internet	Can serve a wide role from personal information transmission to group sessions to blogging.
Mobile phones	Deliver timely, short information. Supportive role. Provide access to internet sources.

In the 1970s, several large-scale community health promotion trials involving the mass media were carried out. Three of the best known were the North Karelia project in Finland (Puska et al. 1985), the North Coast Health Lifestyle Program in Australia (Egger, Donovan & Spark 1993), and the Stanford three- and five-city studies in the US (Maccoby et al. 1977). These trials generally involved comparing control communities with mass media only interventions and mass media plus community-based programs. The general conclusion from these studies was that maximum change is best achieved through the combination of mass media and community-based programs, but that mass media alone can have some impact, albeit limited. For example, road safety advertising and publicity alone can raise awareness of an issue, and may even result in a minor short-term behaviour change. However, without concurrent visible enforcement activities, any behavioural effect may be shortlived. At the same time, the impact of enforcement activities appears to be enhanced by accompanying advertising and publicity (Elder et al. 2004; Tay 2005).

The effectiveness of the media, either alone or as a contributing element in health promotion and injury prevention campaigns, has been confirmed in a number of different areas across the globe. This is particularly so in relation to HIV/AIDS interventions, tobacco control, road safety, sun protection, physical activity and general health promotion, injury prevention, racism prevention, domestic violence prevention, recycling promotion, de-stigmatisation of mental illness and crime prevention (e.g. see Cavill & Bauman 2004; Dawson 2009; Donovan & Vlais 2005; Elder et al. 2004; Hornik 2002; Lannon 2008; Sartorius & Schulze 2005; Singhal et al. 2004; Tay 2005). As with many areas, where the mass media have failed, it is not so much that mass media are ineffective, but rather the message has been poor, the targeting ineffective, the objectives unrealistic or the evaluation inappropriate. Where campaigns have been based on sound social and cognitive models, where community activities are included, and where all the principles of social marketing and health promotion are integrated, the results have been positive. Also, unrealistic objectives are often set for the media. It is unrealistic, for example, to expect that advertising alone will have a significant impact on a man's violent behaviour—but it can have a substantial influence on encouraging a violent man to seek help for his behaviour (Donovan & Vlais 2005; Donovan, Paterson & Francas 1999).

Mass media methods

Donovan and Henley (2010) present a two-dimensional framework for media methods and channels:

* five major media *methods:* advertising (including sponsorship), publicity (including public relations and infonews), edutainment, civic journalism and word-of-mouth (including through social media)
* four major types of *channels* through which messages are delivered to target audiences: broadcast, print, newer technologies and social media.

The framework is shown in Figure 6.1, where the number of asterisks represents the degree of applicability of each method for each channel. It can be noted that the newer social media are included as a major channel for delivery of messages via word-of-mouth.

Advertising

Advertising is the paid placement of messages in various media vehicles by an identified source. Hence advertising includes tools such as sponsorship and product placement. Advertising also includes the voluntary placement by the media of social change messages that are clearly in the form of paid advertisements (called community or public service announcements: CSAs or PSAs).

Publicity

Publicity refers to the unpaid placement of messages in the media, usually in news or current affairs programs, but also in feature articles or documentaries. Publicity involves persuading the media to run a particular story or cover a particular event in a way that creates, maintains or increases the target audience's awareness of or favourable attitudes towards the organisation's

	Main channels			
Main methods	**Broadcast:** TV, radio, cinema	**Print:** newspaper magazines outdoor	**Newer technology:** web, mobiles, iPods	**Social media:** networking, blogs, wikis
Advertising and sponsorship	*****	*****	***	**
Publicity, PR and infonews	****	*****	***	**
Edutainment	*****	*	*	
Civic journalism	*	****	**	*
Word-of-mouth		*	*	****

* Number of asterisks represents the degree of applicability of each method for each channel.

Figure 6.1: A framework for using media in social marketing: methods by channels
Donovan & Henley 2010

products or message, or towards the organisation itself. Many campaigns now involve press conferences with celebrities and staged events, supported by such activities as providing the media with press releases, CDs/DVDs feature articles and photographs, and by making experts available for interview on radio and television.

Infonews

Infonews (Donovan & Henley 2010) is a variation on the usual press release. It refers to the systematic placement of desired messages in news items for a specific period as part of a campaign. Journalists are provided with standard paragraphs that can accompany news about various topics, usually along with a supporting fact sheet (e.g. the CARRS fact sheet featured opposite). For example, reports of road crashes can include closing statements that 'crashes due to fatigue are estimated to constitute up to 30 per cent of road deaths. Fatigue occurs not only on country roads, but in early morning traffic resulting from late nights or disturbed sleep'.

Edutainment

An increasing use of the media for health promotion is the deliberate inclusion of socially desirable messages in entertainment vehicles, such as

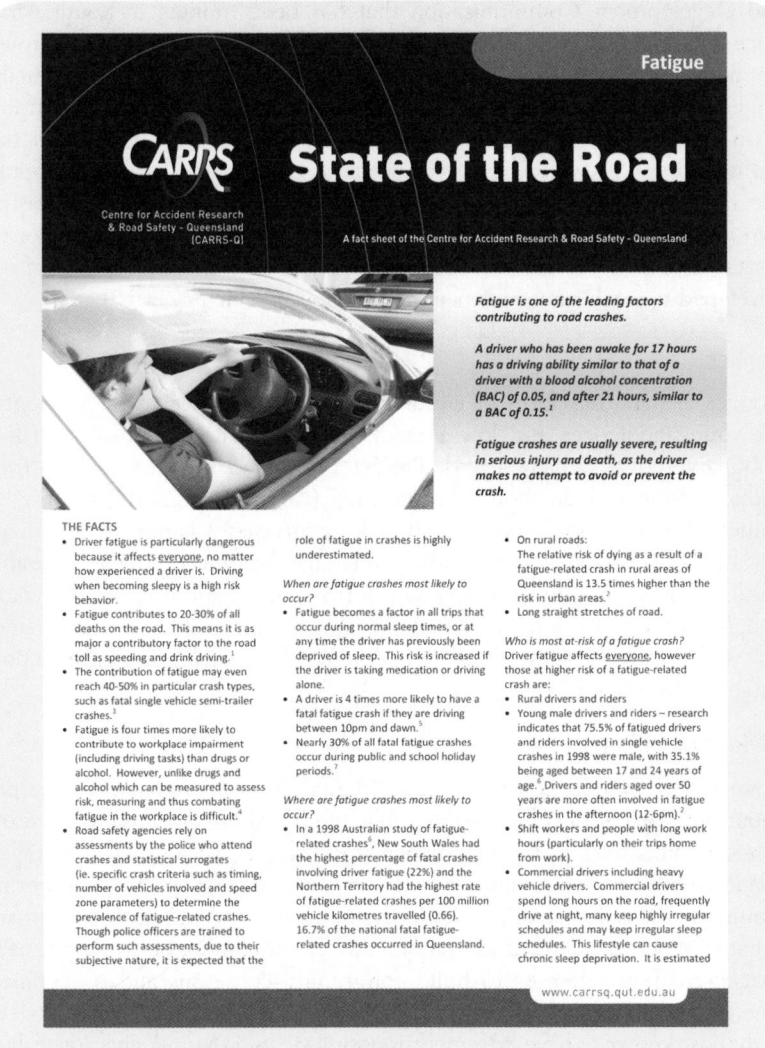

Fact sheet on fatigue and road safety

Queensland Centre for Accident Research and Road Safety

television soap operas, to achieve social change objectives. For example, the Harvard alcohol project in the US asked television writers to introduce into top-rated TV programs actions and themes that would reinforce and encourage a social norm that drivers don't drink (DeJong & Winsten 1990).

Perhaps the most systematic, comprehensive and sustained example is that of *Soul City*, a multimedia edutainment strategy of the Institute for Health

141

and Development Communication that has been running in South Africa since 1992. *Soul City* 'aims to empower people and communities through the power of mass media' (CASE 1997), using television, radio, print media, public relations and advertising, and education packages. *Soul City* (a fictitious town in South Africa) began as a television soap opera, a half-hour drama that ran weekly for 13 weeks. It has reportedly become one of the most popular programs on television and won the Avanti award for excellence in broadcasting two years in succession in the 1990s. The original radio drama component consisted of 45 × 15-minute episodes (in eight different languages) and was developed to reach rural audiences (see Donovan & Henley 2010).

Comics

Comics are another form of edutainment that have been widely adopted for young audiences and low literacy, lesser educated populations (Beck 2006; Everett & Schaay 1994). Project Northland includes a *Slick Tracy* comic dealing with alcohol and drug issues (Komro et al. 2004) and the US National Youth Anti-Drug Program also incorporates comic strip formats. Until 2007, Streetwize was a leading Australian communicator of accessible, culturally relevant and entertaining information on social issues for young people outside the school system via the medium of comic magazines. Its work can be viewed at www.powerhousemuseum.com/collection/database/?irn=366524.

Civic journalism

Rosen (1994) describes civic (or public) journalism as: 'an unfolding philosophy about the place of the journalist in public life [that] has emerged most clearly in recent initiatives in the newspaper world that show journalists trying to connect with their communities . . . by encouraging civic participation or re-grounding the coverage of politics in the imperatives of public discussion and debate'. Whereas standard journalism thrives on conflict and disagreement, civic journalism attempts to build community consensus and cooperation; where standard journalism seeks to emphasise differences and seek interviews with those known to have extremely opposing views on a topic, civic journalism emphasises similarities and seeks to emphasise more moderate views.

Word-of-mouth

In the commercial arena, word-of-mouth advertising generally refers to people passing on favourable or unfavourable reports on a product to others; diffusion models have always considered such interpersonal exchanges an important component of how readily an innovation is adopted. While marketers sometimes tried to hurry this process along by sampling promotions and developing advertising materials that generated discussion, the advent of the internet and social network media has provided a whole new dimension to the concept. Feedback on products is now all over the net, with comments on such things as new movies instantly sent around the world. Donovan and Henley (2010) list three major changes in this area:

- The speed with which information spreads by word-of-mouth means it can reach millions of people all around the globe.
- Companies now make ads specifically to be spread via word-of-mouth (via YouTube or simply email) ('buzz campaigns' or 'viral marketing').
- 'Stealth marketing' (not disclosing one's identity as a marketer in a communication), 'shilling' (paying someone to endorse a product without disclosing that fact) and 'infiltration' (using a fake identity in an online discussion) appear to be increasing as marketers become aware of the potential import of social media.

CASE STUDY **6.1**

Civic journalism—the *Akron Beacon Journal*'s race relations project

Following race riots in Los Angeles, the *Akron Beacon Journal* instituted a year-long series of articles, entitled 'A Question of Color', dealing with five issues: racial attitudes, housing, education, economic status and crime. Each topic was presented over three or four consecutive days, covering several pages each day, and including a number of graphics and people photos. The amount of space devoted to the series was a clear indicator to the reader of the importance placed on the issue by the newspaper.

The articles contained a mix of statistical information (e.g. percentage of home ownership by colour, percentage occupational status by colour), traditional journalism reporting and interpretation of past and current events, the identification of major changes and non-changes over the decades, reports on the results of focus groups among both blacks and whites that probed beliefs and attitudes held by the two groups towards each other (and post-group interviews with participants), and reports on survey research of the extent to which people in the community held various beliefs and attitudes. Right from the start, the journal's readers were invited to 'Tell us what you think' about race relations and 'how blacks and whites can better understand each other', by faxing, phoning or writing to the newspaper. The newspaper periodically printed readers' contributions. This involvement of the community evolved into the 'Coming Together' community project, which continued after the 'A Question of Color' series finished in December 1993.

Donovan & Henley 2010

Donovan and Henley (2010) report a number of attempts to use viral marketing in health promotion and social marketing. For example, the 'Nicomarket' viral component of the European HELP tobacco control campaign, aimed at young people aged 18–24 years, featured a series of eight videos developed for the internet. These promoted ironically branded products to highlight the short-term negative impacts of smoking (such as 'Smoke' perfume, 'Nicoteeth' toothpaste, 'Nicoclean' face cleanser and 'Nicobreeze' air freshener). Each video featured a 'share with friends' email function. The website was launched in Europe in October 2007 with banner advertising on key target group websites (including MSN, Yahoo, Meetic and TillLate). The videos were also posted on key external sites with high youth visitation, such as MTV, DailyMotion, YouTube and Metacafe. In its first year the Nicomarket website registered more than 291 000 visits, with 13 per cent of viewers forwarding the link on to others. The videos posted on external sites were also viewed 3.5 million times within the first two months (Hastings et al. 2008).

Websites, interactive information technology and social media

The internet has increased the average individual's access to information, and, for certain marketers, has provided a sales channel to reach markets far beyond their small geographic catchment areas. However, it has not increased the public's ability to interpret information, or to judge the reliability and validity of the information provided. This unfettered access to the web increases the need for credible pro-social organisations to not only have a strong presence on the web but to also continue to position themselves in the public eye as the credible, authoritative sources for information in their areas.

CASE STUDY **6.2**

Interactive websites: the US National Youth Anti-Drug Media Campaign

This campaign brings together a number of interactive websites aimed at youth, parents, teachers, media personnel and other stakeholders, placing messages on a variety of partners' websites, placing advertising on consumer websites and with a major internet service provider (AOL, America On Line), and developing messages and programs for leading child and parent news content sites. One partnership includes a deal with Marvel Comic Books that produces a special Spider-Man comic book series (downloadable from the web) teaching kids anti-drug messages and media literacy skills for deconstructing what they see and hear in movies, television and popular songs.

Schwartz 2000; from Donovan & Henley 2010

For health promoters, the web provides a relatively efficient and inexpensive forum for the development and dissemination of interventions and materials. For example, the website of the Communication Initiative Network (www.comminit.com) provides links to sites under several themes including early childhood development, HIV/AIDS, entertainment education, information and communication technologies, natural resource management and polio. There is a wealth of information from around the globe under all of these themes, including news reports, updates and evaluations. The site also provides information on broad topics such as change theories, online research planning models and strategic thinking. There is a global site, as well as a Spanish-language Latin American site and an English-language African site, each with its own themes.

Multimedia and interactive technology developments are present on many websites, particularly those targeting children and youth. One of the most popular interactive concepts is that of making choices at various decision points in a narrative, which then lead to very different outcomes as the story unfolds. This can be done with live actors on the stage taking directions from the audience, in books or on DVDs or websites. For example, in August 2009 the World Anti-Doping Agency (WADA) released two 'choose your own adventure' books by Ramsey Montgomery, one, targeting 8–12 year olds, deals with cheating issues (*Always Picked Last*), and the other, for older athletes, deals with the use of performance-enhancing substances and supplements (*Track Star!*). Most opportunities for interactivity are via websites and DVDs/CDs, although digital interactive TV and radio are becoming widespread.

Many health organisations have developed interactive websites where visitors can, for example, answer a questionnaire regarding their dietary habits and receive an immediate 'diagnosis' and 'prognosis' re dietary changes. Anti-tobacco campaigners have developed similar methods that classify smokers according to their stage of change, and then present messages 'tailored' to the smoker's stage of change and other characteristics (Borland, Balmford & Hunt 2004). The 'Act–Belong–Commit' mental health promotion campaign (www.actbelongcommit.org.au) includes a self-assessment tool along with a 'discovery' tool that directs an individual to activities they might be interested in that could boost their mental health.

Mobile phones

Mobile phone ownership is growing rapidly. The International Telecommunication Union (2011) estimates that at the end of 2011, there were 5.9 billion mobile subscriptions, equivalent to 87 per cent of the world population (and 79% in the developing world). Text messaging of health-related information is becoming common as a component of health campaigns, for example, reminding British women to take their contraceptive pill, encouraging Australian AIDS patients to comply with their medication

145

regimens and encouraging African-Americans to text STI questions to the San Francisco Health Department (Zimmerman 2007). Many health interventions now include a mobile app as part of their communication strategies (see the Act–Belong–Commit app). In addition to education and awareness initiatives, observers see five further areas of mobiles application: remote data collection, remote monitoring, communication and training for healthcare workers, disease and epidemic outbreak tracking, and diagnostic and treatment support (Donovan & Henley 2010).

Games

Games have been developed as part of health promotion interventions; it has been shown that they can increase knowledge and impact on behaviour (Bandura 2004). For example, *Packy & Marlon*, an interactive videogame designed to improve self-care among children and adolescents with diabetes, was evaluated in a 6-month randomised controlled trial. In the game, players take the role of animated characters who manage their diabetes by monitoring blood glucose, taking insulin injections and choosing foods, while setting out to save a diabetes summer camp from marauding rats and mice who have stolen the diabetes supplies. The *Packy & Marlon* game players showed significant improvements over the control group in terms of diabetes-related self-efficacy, communication with parents about diabetes and self-care behaviours, and a decrease in unscheduled urgent doctor visits (Brown et al. 1997). The latest variation on such games are Wii 'exergames' with the Nintendo Wii selling more than 11 million consoles in the US from late 2006 to mid-2008 (Anders 2008). There is also Wii Fit (a wired balance board leads players through 40 different exercises), Konami DanceDance Revolution (uses a mat, screen and music), the Sony Playstation Eye and Cateye Fitness GameBike (a stationary bike that links to other gaming consoles and allows the player to control the game by pedalling and steering the bike), and no doubt many more by the time of publication.

While research on these exergames' health and fitness benefits is limited, they do appear to provide positive behavioural and psychological effects in that people enjoy them, and they maintain higher adherence rates than traditional exercise equipment (Mark & Rhodes 2009).

Social media

Social media can be defined as electronic tools, technologies and applications that facilitate interactive communication and content exchange, with the distinct feature that the user can easily alternate between audience and author (Donovan & Henley 2010). Types of social media include blogs, forums, virtual worlds, wikis and social networks (see box opposite). Their key characteristics are participation and connection. As noted above, it is now commonplace for health promoters to have a social media presence. For example, the US Centers for Disease Control and Prevention (CDC) has a presence on Twitter, Facebook, MySpace, DailyStrength, its own YouTube channel, Flickr site and iTune podcasts and Second Life Island—in addition to offering online videos, podcasts, RSS feeds and widgets on the CDC website. CDC used all these media in its comprehensive education and awareness campaign about swine flu (novel H1N1 flu), the pandemic that swept the globe in 2009 (Donovan & Henley 2010).

Examples of current social media sites

Blogs
Image/video sharing sites: Flickr, YouTube
Internet forums
Microblogs: Twitter, Plurk
Mobile websites
Podcasts
Professional networking: LinkedIn
RSS feeds
Social bookmarking: Del.icio.us
Social-networking sites: Facebook, Myspace
Social news: Digg
Virtual worlds: Second Life, Whyville
Widgets
Wikis

Donovan and Henley (2010) note that while health promoters are enthusiastically embracing these new social media, their actual and relative impact and effectiveness have not been established to date. They warn that their use must be carefully considered alongside other media in terms of what target audiences we wish to reach and impact, what sort of messages we want to send, and what are our communication and behaviour objectives. As political campaigns both in the US (Abrom & Lefebvre 2009) and Australia (MacNamara & Bell 2008) have shown, social media have a role. President Barack Obama's 2012 campaign in particular demonstrates the capacity of social media to mobilise supporters and to raise funds, which were then spent to great effect in the traditional media, particularly television.

Choosing media methods

The decision about whether to use advertising, publicity, edutainment, civic journalism or word-of-mouth (including through social media) or some combination of these in a health promotion campaign is determined by a number of factors: the objectives of the campaign, the budget, the relative effectiveness of the different methods in reaching and influencing the target audiences, the complexity of the message, time constraints, relations with the media, and the nature and types of media and media vehicles available.

From the campaign manager's perspective, the primary advantages of paid advertising relate to control factors: that is, control over message content and exposure (timing and location), and hence target audience and frequency of exposure. Control over message content not only allows precise specification of the informational content of the message but also allows the creation of imagery and the use of various message executional techniques and appeals that enhance the persuasive power of the message. Advertising's major disadvantage is cost. However, because the number of people exposed to advertising is usually quite large, the cost per individual contact and impact is often low, especially relative to face-to-face methods.

Publicity shares the ability of advertising to reach large numbers of people in a relatively short period of time, but has the disadvantage of less control over message content, message exposure and frequency (unless the issue is sufficiently newsworthy to attract continuing coverage for several days). A press release, for example, might be rewritten in a way that omits or distorts crucial information, be relegated to the later pages of a newspaper, appear only in a very late TV or radio news spot, or even be totally ignored. On the other hand, publicity is generally perceived as more credible than paid advertising (because the source is presumably unbiased or less biased) and is less costly. However, costs are incurred in developing materials, staging events and so on, and often there are fees for engaging professional public relations agencies.

Edutainment also has the ability to reach large numbers of people in a relatively short period of time, but has the disadvantages of reduced control over message content. The primary advantage of edutainment is the ability to attract the attention of people who might otherwise deliberately avoid messages that appear in an obvious educational form. Where a health authority or sponsoring body is not directly involved in producing the show, edutainment can be done economically. If a show is a commercial success, the health organisation could even earn a profit (Coleman & Meyer 1990).

Websites are now an expected part of any health promotion initiative. Useful websites allow the audience access to information about an issue and allow stakeholders access to program information. Interactive elements can be built into the site, as well as links to other sites and to social media such as Facebook and YouTube. Website design becomes expensive when interactive elements are included, but the major issues are maintaining and updating the site. Sites are often established in a burst of enthusiasm but are quickly neglected and become dated.

Civic journalism is useful for complex issues that require extensive information to be absorbed in a non-emotive atmosphere. The major difficulty in Australia is that there is no established tradition of civic journalism; mass circulation newspapers and television channels appear to be focused on advertising revenue rather than on quality journalism, and hence individual journalists have little support from their editors and publishers (Donovan & Henley 2010).

Roles of the media in health promotion campaigns

There appear to be three major roles, two of which primarily apply to targeting individual risky behaviour change and one to achieving socio-political objectives.

Targeting individual behaviour change

According to Donovan (1991), the two primary communication objectives for most campaigns are to inform (or educate) and to persuade (or motivate). The distinction between these two roles is blurred in that the provision of information is generally not intended for its own sake, but is usually meant to lead to desired behaviour changes. However, although information alone can arouse emotions and motivate some people to cease an unhealthy practice, it is clear from the public health literature that information by itself is insufficient to bring about desired behaviour changes in most risk behaviours for most individuals.

Targeting socio-political change—media advocacy

Most uses of the mass media in health promotion have been directed towards changing risk behaviours at the individual level. However, the mass media are also used to advocate for socio-political environmental changes that affect health (Chapman & Lupton 1994). Advocacy for health promotion is a relatively ill-defined process with broad general characteristics, summed up by Chapman (2004) as being:

1. a focus on 'upstream' goals
2. goals that are invariably contested
3. methods that are opportunistic and responsive.

The quit smoking lobby is to date the most professional health advocacy group successfully using media advocacy. It has used the media to redefine smoking as a public health issue of concern to all, and to attack the morals and motives of tobacco companies' marketing techniques. The subsequent arousal of public opinion has been used to support direct lobbying of legislative changes, such as restricting the advertising of cigarettes and the sponsorship of sporting and arts events by tobacco companies. Advocacy often has as its primary outcome a change in the physical environment (e.g. protests for better roads). However, in achieving such an outcome, it generally aims initially at changing the socio-cultural environment. Other areas in which advocacy has worked effectively are drink-driving, sports injury prevention, HIV/AIDS control and nutrition advertising, giving rise to several publications that outline processes and practices of advocacy (Wallack et al. 1993; Chapman 2007; Siegal & Doner 2007).

Figure 6.2 shows that each of these objectives can be pursued via all of the available media methods, although as the number of asterisks indicate, some methods are potentially more effective than others for some objectives.

Main methods	Objectives		
	Educate (Inform)	Motivate (Persuade)	Advocate (Policy change)
Advertising and sponsorship	***	*****	**
Publicity, PR and infonews	***	**	***
Edutainment	***	***	***
Civic journalism	*****	***	****
Word-of-mouth	***	***	****

* Number of asterisks represents the effectiveness of methods for each objective.

Figure 6.2: Using media in social marketing: methods by objectives

Donovan & Henley 2010

Both individual and socio-political change objectives should be combined for any comprehensive health campaign. However, in some cases, campaigns targeted at individuals must first have some broader social influence on beliefs and attitudes towards the recommended behaviour before political advocacy objectives can be achieved. For example, it is unlikely that efforts to frame smoking as a public health issue would have been as successful without prior Quit campaigns that emphasised the ill-health effects of smoking. Similarly, efforts to control smoking indoors undoubtedly were facilitated by increasing awareness of the health effects of passive smoking.

There are a number of objectives that can be classified under the three overall roles of information, motivation or persuasion and advocacy, which are discussed below in the context of tobacco control. However, it should be noted that the classifications are not mutually exclusive.

Informational objectives

- Informing (or educating) people about the negative health effects of smoking and passive smoking, and the positive health effects of cessation and smokefree areas.
- Clarifying misperceptions and/or confusion that people might have about various health effects of smoking.
- Reminding people of the positive and negative health effects of which they are already aware and maintaining the salience of this knowledge.
- Directing people to information on where and how to get help, or how to help themselves.
- Informing the target audience of specific events ('15 June is Quit Day'), or programs and services ('Quit classes, 3 pm daily, St Bernard's Hall').

Motivational or persuasion objectives

- Reinforcing non-smokers or ex-smokers, especially recent quitters.
- Generating emotional arousal to increase people's motivations to quit smoking.
- Sensitising or predisposing individuals to other contributory influences (arguably the major role as a facilitator of behaviour change), such as family pressures to quit or availability of assistance to quit.
- Increasing awareness of both prescriptive and, where appropriate, popular norms (Cialdini 1984), and hence providing social support for those who wish to quit.
- Stimulating word-of-mouth communications about the health issues in question and hence encouraging peer (and other) group discussion and decision making—a very important role for the diffusion of social issues, including in social media.

Advocacy-related objectives

- Increasing community awareness of smoking as a public health issue; that is, placing the issue on the community's agenda, or 'agenda setting'.

- Creating or increasing community awareness of a particular point of view with respect to passive smoking; that is, framing the community agenda.
- Creating or maintaining a favourable attitude towards such issues as restrictions on tobacco promotion and providing smokefree entertainment venues.
- Creating a view that the issue is a sufficiently serious one for community concern; that is, legitimising the issue.
- Generating a positive community mood within which health authority policies—including research and regulatory measures, such as banning of sponsorship by tobacco companies and introducing plain packaging—can be introduced with minimal opposition and/or maximal support.

Components of successful media campaigns

A number of researchers, both in health promotion and in communications, have attempted to identify the conditions under which use of media is most effective in promoting health. Distilling a number of reviews and other research leads to the following practical recommendations for designing a successful campaign:

- *Carry out formative research*—intuition is not a sufficient basis on which to devise a campaign. Materials should be developed from skilled formative research (i.e. focus groups, surveys), pre-tested and evaluated during exposure.
- *Base the campaign on a model of attitude–behaviour change*—those discussed in Chapter 2 are most relevant for health promotion.
- *Fully understand the topic being communicated*—some topics are difficult and complex to teach (e.g. the nature of drugs and their effects), whereas others might be easily communicated (e.g. hygiene). Similarly, certain well-established types of behaviour are difficult to change (e.g. smoking), whereas others require only a minor effort (e.g. not littering).
- *Use skilled creative personnel*—determining a message is simple. Executing that message in a way that is optimally received and acted upon by a target audience is a highly skilled process.
- *Understand the audience*—the extent to which a message is attended to, comprehended and used by an audience is largely determined by the extent to which the messenger understands the audience. Detailed profiles of an audience need to be established as a preliminary to media development if a message is to be optimally received.

- *Target the message*—different subgroups have different needs, interests, beliefs and attitudes. Hence, different messages—or at least different message executions—should be tailored to different groups. Different groups can be reached through different channels.
- *Take account of interpersonal and peer influences*—campaigns should attempt to stimulate interpersonal contact, such as the promotion of group and community activities and the activation of interpersonal communication networks—including social media networks.
- *Optimise contact with the message*—this doesn't mean total bombardment. Research indicates that concentrated bursts of spot messages often work better than the same quantity of messages strung out over a long period.
- *Use multiple channels*—multiple communication channels (i.e. different media and media vehicles plus various non-media channels) tend to have a synergistic effect, are mutually reinforcing and can carry different types of information.
- *Use a credible source or spokesperson*—source credibility is a major factor affecting message acceptance. Spokespersons are often assumed to be credible to the target audience, for example, the use of celebrities and sport stars in anti-drug promotions to youth is common practice, yet research suggests that youth identify only with certain aspects of an idealised role model, such as their ability to play music or sport. If other aspects (e.g. their attitude to drugs) conflict with overwhelming peer pressure, the model will be discarded rather than the antisocial habit. Testing source credibility is essential in pretesting the message.
- *Set realistic goals and a realistic duration for the study*—major shifts in behaviour are not common in large populations over short periods. Hence it is important that intermediate goals, such as knowledge and attitudinal changes, are set rather than behavioural goals. Also, ongoing campaigns are necessary to maintain awareness and to reinforce attitude and behaviour change. Furthermore, many campaigns set large, unrealistic changes as their criteria for success (e.g. reducing alcoholism) rather than more realistic immediate changes (e.g. reducing drink-driving).
- *Provide environmental supports for change*—research has shown consistently that most media campaigns require 'on-the-ground' backup support for optimum effect. To accomplish this, media should be accompanied by strategies of community organisation.
- *Ensure that input from a behavioural scientist guides the communications agency*—commercial agencies need to be guided by behavioural science principles. The danger otherwise is that creative ideas will drive the strategy rather than the strategy driving the creative ideas.

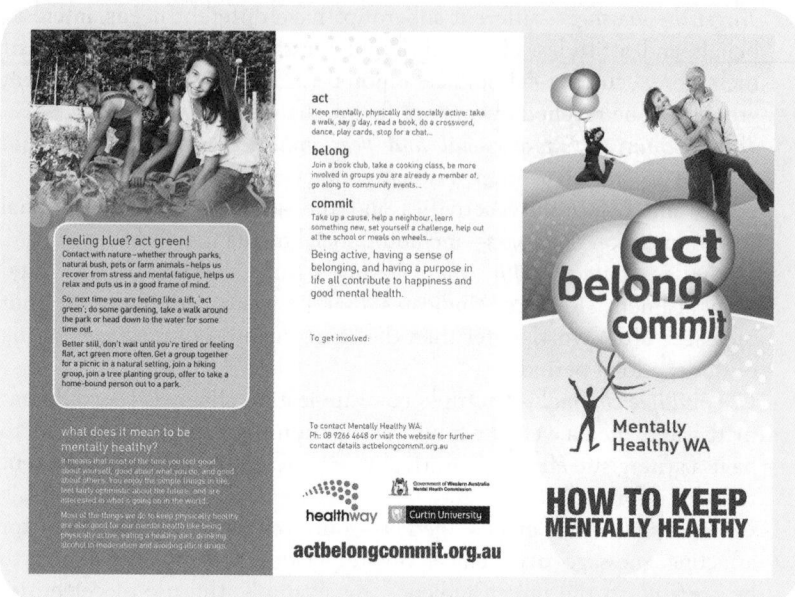

The 'Feeling Blue? Act Green!' Act–Belong–Commit ad's catchy headline encourages time spent in natural settings and a concern for the environment as ways to promote mentally healthy behaviours

Courtesy of the Act-Belong-Commit campaign coordinated by Mentally Healthy WA

Appropriate situations for media use

Some of the situations in which mass and targeted media have been found to be most appropriate are:

- *When wide exposure is desired*—mass media offer the widest possible exposure, although this might be at some cost. Cost–benefit considerations therefore are at the core of media selection.
- *When the timeframe is urgent*—mass media offer the best opportunity for reaching either large numbers of people or specific target groups within a short timeframe.
- *When public discussion is likely to facilitate the educational process*—media messages can be emotional and thought provoking. Because of the possible breadth of coverage, intrusion can occur at many different levels, stimulating discussion and thereby expanding the influence of a message.
- *When awareness is a main goal*—by their very nature the media are tools for awareness creating. Where awareness of a health issue is important to the resolution of that issue, the mass media can increase awareness quickly and effectively.

- *When media authorities are 'on side'*—where journalists, editors and programmers are 'on side' with respect to a particular health issue, this often guarantees greater support in terms of space and editorial content.

Hard-to-reach audiences

Some criticism of the use of mass media has centred on the claim that mass media are ineffective in reaching important target groups. In some cases this is a valid criticism in that media campaigns have been directed towards various groups that would have been more effectively targeted via some other method. The question remains whether the media can be used to reach 'hard-to-reach' groups and, if so, what roles would they play for these groups?

Hard-to-reach groups are usually defined in terms of their non-responsiveness to mainstream media campaigns. However, it is important to distinguish between those who are hard to reach because of (1) low access to mainstream media, and those who are hard to reach because of (2) apparent imperviousness to media campaigns. The latter definition is the most used, and accessibility is often included as a correlate of personality and lifestyle factors, such as a distrust of large government organisations, a sense of fatalism and poor cognitive processing skills. We suggest two alternative definitions:

1. *hard-to-reach*—to refer to those not accessible via media
2. *hard-to-influence*—to refer to those not responsive to messages delivered via the media.

Groups like sex workers, intravenous drug users, street kids and other homeless people, Aboriginal fringe dwellers and non-English-speaking immigrants are generally thought of with respect to accessibility. Yet there is now considerable evidence that such groups are accessible via various media, including ethnic media, although care must be taken in scheduling and vehicle selection.

With respect to both accessibility and responsiveness, the answer lies in carrying out adequate formative research to assess, first, whether a potential target audience is accessible and then, given accessibility, whether it is likely to be responsive to media messages. In some cases, the role of the media might be limited to directing people to other campaign interventions (e.g. telephone information services, interpreter services, needle exchange locations) rather than to belief or attitude change.

Concluding comments

The effective application of these media methods for health promotion requires close cooperation between media experts, marketing experts, health professionals and behavioural scientists with expertise in communication theory and attitude and behaviour change. For example, the Australian Government's first major national tobacco campaign was directed by a special advisory group (headed by a behavioural scientist), and included health promotion, social marketing and consumer behaviour experts, all with considerable experience in tobacco control.

When considering various media channels, some points to remember are:

* When it comes to media, new does not always mean better—it is the end (the goal) that counts, not the means (the channel).
* Strategy should drive creativity—not the other way around.
* We are social beings; social networking is not new. What is new are the opportunities for non–face-to-face networking on a grand scale with 'virtual friends'.

Finally, Donovan and Henley (2010) note that cyber networking may decline as people miss the human contact of face-to-face interactions. This is evident in some areas where people name their cyber chat room 'fireside chats' in what appears to be an attempt to generate some 'warmth' in the interactions. Others are reviving the old concept of meeting face-to-face in cafes to talk about societal issues—informing each other about place, time and topic by . . . social media of course!

References

Abroms, L., & Lefebvre, R., 2009, Obama's wired campaign: lessons for public health communication, *J Health Communications* 14:415–23.

Anders, M., 2008, As good as the real thing? *ACE FitnessMatters* July/August:7–9.

Bandura, A., 2004, Health promotion by social cognitive means, *Health Educ Behav* 312:143–64.

Beck, R., 2006, Popular media for HIV/AIDS prevention? Comparing two comics: Kingo and the Sara Communication Initiative, *J Mod African Stud* 44(r4):513–41.

Borland, R., Balmford, J., & Hunt, D., 2004, The effectiveness of personally tailored computer-generated advice letters for smoking cessation, *Addiction* 99(3):369–77.

Brown, S., Lieberman, D., Gemeny, B., Fan, Y., Wilson, D., & Pasta, D., 1997, Educational video game for juvenile diabetes: results of a controlled trial, *Informatics for Health and Social Care* 22(1):77–89.

Cavill, N., & Bauman, A., 2004, Changing the way people think about health-enhancing physical activity: do mass media campaigns have a role? *J Sports Sci*, 22(8):771–90.

CASE (Community Agency for Social Enquiry), 1997, *Let the Sky Be the Limit: Soul City Evaluation Report*, Braamfontein, South Africa.

Chapman, S., 2004, Public health advocacy, in Moodie, R., & Hulme, A. (Eds), *Hands-on Health Promotion*, IP Communications, Melbourne.

Chapman, S., 2007, *Public Health Advocacy and Tobacco Control: Making Smoking History*, Blackwell, Oxford.

Chapman, S., & Lupton, D., 1994, *The Fight for Public Health: Principles and Practice of Media Advocacy*, BMJ Publishing Group, London.

Cialdini, R.B., 1984, *Influence*, Quill, New York.

Coleman, P.L., & Meyer, R.C. (Eds), 1990, *Proceedings from the Enter-Educate Conference: Entertainment for Social Change*, Johns Hopkins University Center for Communication Programs, Baltimore.

Dawson, N. (Ed), 2009, *Advertising Works 17: Proving the Payback on Marketing Investment*, World Advertising Research Center, Oxfordshire.

DeJong, W., & Winsten, J.A., 1990, The use of mass media in substance abuse prevention, *Health Affairs* Summer:30–46.

Donovan, R.J., 1991, Public health advertising: execution guidelines for health promotion professionals, *Health Promot J Aust* 1:40–5.

Donovan, R.J., & Henley, N., 2010, *Social Marketing: An International Perspective*, Cambridge University Press, Cambridge.

Donovan, R.J., Paterson, D., & Francas, M., 1999, Targeting male perpetrators of intimate partner violence: Western Australia's 'Freedom from Fear' campaign, *Soc Marketing Quarterly* 5(3), 127–43.

Donovan, R., & Vlais, R., 2005, *A Review of Communication Components of Anti-Racism and Pro Diversity Social Marketing/Public Education Campaigns*, Report to VicHealth, Melbourne.

Egger, G., Donovan, R.J., & Spark, R., 1993, *Health and the Media: Principles and Practice for Health Promotion*, McGraw-Hill, Sydney.

Elder, R., Shults, R., Sleet, D., Nichols, J., Thompson, R., & Rajab, W., 2004, Effectiveness of mass media campaigns for reducing drinking and driving and alcohol-involved crashes: a systematic review, *Am J Prev Med* 27(1):57–65.

Everett, K., & Schaay, N., 1994, Country watch: South Africa, *AIDS Health Promot Exchange* 1:7–8.

Hastings, G., Freeman, J., Spackove, R., & Siquier, P., 2008, HELP: A European public health brand in the making, in Evans, D.W., & Hastings, G. (Eds), *Public Health Branding: Applying Marketing for Social Change*, Oxford University Press.

Hornick, R., 2002, *Public Health Communication: Evidence for Behavioural Change* Lawrence Erlbaum, New Jersey.

International Telecommunication Union, 2011, *The world in 2011—ICT facts and figures*, ITU, Geneva.

Komro, K., Perry, C., Veblen-Mortenson, S., Bosma, L., Dudovitz, B., Williams, C., Jones-Webb, R., & Toomey, T., 2004, Brief report: the adaptation of Project Northland for urban youth, *J Pediatric Psychol* 29(6):457–66.

Lannon, J. (Ed), 2008, *How Public Service Advertising Works*, World Advertising Research Center, Oxfordshire.

Maccoby, N., Farquhar, J., Wood, P.D., & Alexander, J., 1977, Reducing the risk of cardiovascular disease: effects of a community-based campaign on knowledge and behavior, *J Community Health* 3(2):100–14.

Macnamara, J., & Bell, P., 2008, *E-electioneering: Use of New Media in the 2007 Australian Federal Election*, University of Technology, Sydney and Media Monitors.

Manning, N., 2009, The new media communications model: a progress report, in Dawson, N. (Ed), *Advertising Works 17: Proving the Payback on Marketing Investment*, IPA/WARC, London.

Mark, R., & Rhodes, R., 2009, Active video games: a good way to exercise, *WellSpring*, 20(4).

Puska, P., Toumilehto, J., Salonen, J., Neittaanmaki, L., Maki, J., & Virtamo, J., 1985, The community based strategy to prevent heart disease: conclusions of the ten years of the North Karelia Project, *Ann Rev Public Health* 6:147–93.

Rosen, J., 1994, Public journalism: first principles, in Rosen, J., & Merritt Jr, D. (Eds), *Public Journalism: Theory and Practice*, Kettering Foundation, Dayton.

Sartorius, N., & Schulze, H., 2005, *Reducing the Stigma of Mental Illness*, Cambridge University Press, Cambridge.

Schwartz, B., 2000, *Social Marketing Workshop*, Academy for Educational Development, Washington, DC.

Siegel, M., & Doner, L., 2007, *Marketing Public Health: Strategies to Promote Social Change*, Jones and Bartlett, Massachusetts.

Singhal, A., Cody, M., Rogers, E., & Sabido, M., 2004, *Entertainment-Education and social change*, Lawrence Erlbaum, New Jersey.

Tay, R., 2005, Drink driving enforcement and publicity campaigns: are the policy recommendations sensitive to model specification? *Accident Analysis Prevention*, 37(2):259–66.

Wallack, L., Dorfman, L., Jernigan, D., & Themba, M., 1993, *Media Advocacy and Public Health: Power for Prevention*, Sage Publications, Newbury Park, Calif.

Zimmerman, R., 2007, Don't 4get ur pills: text messaging for health, *The Wall Street Journal*, 20 November, http://online.wsj.com/article/SB119551720462598532.html, accessed 19 August 2007.

chapter 7

Focus on populations: community-based approaches

Summary of main points

- The underlying purpose of community-based approaches in health promotion is to empower individuals and communities to gain control over the determinants of their own health.
- Capacity building is a means of empowering individuals, organisations and communities to do this.
- Partnerships are a key component of any successful health promotion program.
- Community organisation is a process of introducing positive changes for health in a community by involving that community in achieving largely predetermined goals.
- Community development involves the community in defining the agenda and changing itself with limited guidance and minimal intervention from outside.
- Without community participation and empowerment of individuals and communities, health promotion interventions are likely to be of limited impact.

The role of community processes

As noted previously, the mass media have been used frequently in health promotion as an 'umbrella' to set community agendas, promote awareness and increase knowledge on health issues, thus facilitating other health promotion program components.

However, mass media methods in health promotion can be seen by some as an imposition on a community by 'experts'—often from outside that community—with supposedly greater understanding of what is 'good' for that community. The questions this raises for public policy in a democratic society are obvious. Externally imposed mass media programs have also attracted the criticism that these do not address the underlying social and economic causes of health problems. They can also overlook the needs, cultures, values, aspirations and priorities of local communities. As Baum (2007) cautions, unless applying a very strong 'equity lens', health promotion can act to increase the differences between groups rather than reduce them, even if they improve population health as a whole. She cites as an example the decline in smoking rates in Australia over the period 1998–2004 and notes that while there was a 9 per cent decline in smoking among the lowest socio-economic quintile over this period, the rate of decline for the highest quintile was 35 per cent.

Social equity and health

The issue of how unequally health can be distributed within communities and among classes within societies has become more evident in recent times due to the work of Sir Michael Marmot and Drs Richard Wilkinson and Kate Pickett, among others. Marmot, after several years of study with the British Civil Service, found that position in the social hierarchy and social support in the work environment strongly influenced an individual's health (Stringhini et al. 2012). Wilkinson & Picket (2010) in their seminal study of social inequality found that a range of health and social issues are worse in societies with greater gaps between the rich and the poor. Several other studies have supported this notion of *relative* rather than *absolute* wealth as being the major influence in health status and some have sought to tease out the dimensions of this. Offer and colleagues (2010), for example, found that economic insecurity, based on a range of measures, has the greatest impact on indices of wellbeing such as obesity.

Egger, Swinburn & Islam (2012) on the other hand, using an inter-country comparison of economic measures of wellbeing (GDP), found that beyond a certain point (defined as a 'sweet spot'), increases in GDP lead to a reversal in health trends in some countries, irrespective of overall wealth. This occurs more frequently in countries where there is greater inequity and a more liberal form of governance with greater emphasis on individualism than in countries with the same level of wealth but more emphasis on 'community'. The development of a process of determining and acting upon inequalities through applying an 'equity lens' has become a focal issue in health development care provision, initiated by the World Health Organization (WHO 1999) and other groups (e.g. see the Wellesley Institute at www.wellesleyinstitute.com/publication/health-promotion-through-an-equity-lens).

Increasing focus on communities

As early as 1990, Thompson and Kinne noted the increasing focus on community in health promotion, which they claimed was due—at least in part—to:

> . . . a growing recognition that behaviour is greatly influenced by the environment in which people live. Proponents of community approaches to behavioural change recognise that local values, norms and behaviour patterns have a significant effect on shaping an individual's attitudes and behaviours. (Thompson & Kinne 1990)

It can be easy for beginning health promotion practitioners to believe that they possess the skills to determine what kind of health promotion programs would be most suitable for any particular population group or community. However, the appropriate approach should be awareness of, and responsiveness to, the needs of the communities to be served.

Part of the dilemma in adopting a community perspective is determining what constitutes a community in contemporary society. In the (not so distant) past a community might have been relatively easy to distinguish, with clear geographic boundaries such as a small rural village or town. Today the boundaries are more blurred. A community may still be people living in a rural or urban environment who share cultural origins. But it may also be a group of people who share some other kind of common bond in terms of values, beliefs or interests. The internet has created virtual communities where people from the next suburb or from distant corners of the globe can be joined together to exchange information.

Because a goal of health promotion is to improve health and quality of life for individuals groups and communities, many contemporary health promotion programs are targeted towards communities where health and social inequities are prevalent. These communities need to gain control of the determinants of their own health for their health status to improve. However, it is these same communities where individuals are often the most disempowered and may lack the confidence that their actions can make a difference to change their lives for the better. Therefore, the health promotion practitioner should begin with an understanding of the role that empowerment plays in health, and ideally develop skills in building empowerment among individuals and communities.

Empowerment has been defined as 'access to, and control over, valued resources' (Katz 1984). This definition emphasises the establishment of an equitable distribution of resources to enable those presently disenfranchised and oppressed to experience a fair share of the power.

The *Ottawa Charter for Health Promotion* (WHO 1986) listed five principles for global health promotion action (see Chapter 11). One of these is to *strengthen community action* to achieve better health. The Charter states:

> Health promotion works through concrete and effective community action in setting priorities, making decisions, planning strategies and implementing them to achieve better health. At the heart of this process is the empowerment of communities, their ownership and control of their own endeavours and destinies. (WHO 1986)

Powerlessness, or lack of control over destiny, has emerged as a broad-based risk factor for disease (as discussed in Chapter 1). Empowerment, although more difficult to evaluate, is also an important influencer of health. Wallerstein (1992), for example, noted that:

> Empowerment education . . . involves people in group efforts to identify their problems, to critically assess social and historical roots of problems, to envision a healthier society, and to develop strategies to overcome obstacles in achieving their goals. Through community participation, people develop new beliefs in their ability to influence their personal and social spheres.

Community empowerment embodies an interactive process of change in which institutions and communities become transformed—as the people who participate in changing them become transformed. Rather than pitting individuals against community and overall societal needs, the community empowerment process focuses on both individual and community change (Wallerstein 2002).

Evaluation of community empowerment programs has presented challenges for program evaluators due to the lack of standardised measures and the problem of finding appropriate indicators of program success. Nevertheless, several published case studies provide reason for optimism in terms of progress in developing such measures (Van Daele et al. 2012; Brandstetter et al. 2012).

Conducting empowerment programs in Indigenous communities often presents even greater challenges given their history of disempowerment. However in an evaluation of an Indigenous Australian family empowerment program across four study settings in Australia's Northern Territory and Queensland between 1998 and 2005, Tsey and colleagues (2010) observed that, even within the context of trans-generational grief and despair resulting from colonisation and other discriminatory government policies over time, the program participants demonstrated enhanced capacity to exert greater control over factors shaping their health and wellbeing.

The importance of community empowerment for health is borne out by studies over the years showing that programs emphasising individual preventive actions do not redress inequalities in health. In general, these studies have ascribed inequalities to the broad area of socioeconomic status (Weatherburn 2012; Mackenbach 2012) or more specifically to 'relative poverty' (Wilkinson & Pickett 2010). A closer analysis of the data (Syme 2003; Marmot 1999; Stringhini et al. 2012) reveals that the higher rates of morbidity and mortality in lower social classes cannot be attributed simply to lack of income. Other, less tangible factors associated with class—such as social support, quality of the social and physical environment and number of social stressors—may need to be considered. It is unlikely that programs targeting individual risk factors alone will impact upon these deeper socioeconomic causes. Furthermore, while not strictly correct in all areas, O'Dowd (2012) states that: 'Efforts to persuade people to follow a healthier lifestyle have worked only for wealthier parts of the population and widened the health inequalities divide.' This emphasises the need to consider health literacy in any community initiatives (see Chapter 3).

As empowerment has increasingly entered mainstream discourse, and empowerment programs are now often considered part of a health promotion practitioner's strategy toolkit, it is worth reviewing the effectiveness of empowerment interventions to improve health. In a review conducted by WHO, Wallerstein (2006) observed that much of the research had focused on the empowerment of socially excluded populations such as women, youth, people at risk for HIV/AIDS and the poor, where evidence of effectiveness is often difficult to determine. However, this review did conclude that the most effective strategies have been those that build on and reinforce authentic participation ensuring autonomy in decision making, sense of community and local bonding, and psychological empowerment of the community members themselves (Wallerstein 2006).

To address this area of growing significance in health promotion, strategies addressing change in communities (both driven from within and from without) have borrowed heavily on other disciplines including social sciences, sociology, social welfare and psychology. These include processes that have been termed community organisation and community development, but are often considered under the broader title of 'community-based approaches' (Bracht 1998). However, before undertaking these processes the health promotion practitioner needs to assess the capacity of the community and its various sub-groups to address its health needs and support changes where appropriate to strengthen this capacity.

The elements necessary for social change

Changes in health often require a social movement. Social movements in turn occur when a number of elements come together. These include a number of factors discussed by different writers (Kersh & Morone 2002; Brownell 2004) and modified for presentation here:

1. *An acknowledged crisis (or cause)*—little attention is paid to health issues until these morph into an obvious 'crisis', and particularly one which is felt personally.
2. *A critical mass of scientific evidence*—vested interests will continue to complain about 'lack of evidence', until this becomes overwhelming. At least

continued

163

continued

> 50 000 papers on the dangers of smoking had been published before cigarette manufacturers stopped being proactive about smoking.
> 3. *The obvious presence of victims*—whether real or perceived, the injustice felt when victims are seen to be suffering is crucial to the mobilisation of opposition forces.
> 4. *A tug at the heart strings*—according to Brownell (2004): 'If there is any possibility for major social action and policy change, scientists cannot enforce it and health leaders cannot mandate it. The public must demand it.' Emotional involvement is the key to this happening. Emotions are most strongly aroused when children are seen to be victims.
> 5. *Strong (political) leadership*—only when strong leaders are prepared to resist the influence of powerful vested interests can a significant move be made towards social action. Whether this leads or follows other changes, however, may vary according to circumstance.
> 6. *A balanced perspective*—although vested interests can often be seen as total 'villains', most of these include ordinary people caught up in trying to make a living. Interest groups and even corporations should be encouraged where positive actions are taken to benefit communities, although they may well be criticised when these actions have negative consequences.
>
> In contemporary society, social media can also fan the flames of any social movement by instantly transmitting the movement's messages around the globe—when such messages go viral.

Capacity building

Capacity building is a process of facilitating people and communities to manage their own health.

> Capacity building has been defined as being (at least) three activities: (1) building infrastructure to deliver health promotion programs, (2) building partnerships and organisational environments so that programs are sustained—and health gains are sustained; and (3) building problem-solving capability. (Hawe et al. 2001)

Capacity building not only assists communities to help themselves to scarce resources, but empowers individuals (Eade 1997). This is based on the notion, expressed earlier, that much ill-health stems from social inequality, a sense of helplessness and discrimination or inability to access basic resources. According to Arole, Fuller & Deutschmann (2004):

> Through the processes of information training, and imparting medical, economic, and social skills, individuals and communities gain in self-esteem and self-confidence, and come to realise that they have the capacity within themselves to determine their own lives.

VicHealth's experience over several decades has led it to identify four levels of capacity building for health promotion: individual, community, organisational and system capacity building. Table 7.1 shows examples highlighting each of these levels taken from three of VicHealth's areas of work: tobacco control, mental health and wellbeing, and physical activity.

Table 7.1 Examples highlighting the levels of capacity building

Projects addressing	Smoking rates	Mental health and wellbeing	Physical activity levels
Individual capacity	An individual's knowledge about smoking and employee rights is substantially increased and employees feel able to ask their colleagues not to smoke around them.	Melbourne's Horn-of-Africa communities form a group to address the challenges of settling in a new country. Members build their personal networks and their own skills in addressing issues (that may affect their mental health) such as employment.	Capacity of individual staff members from a local government area (LGA) is increased through VicHealth training and funding. VicHealth builds capacity for program delivery.
Community capacity	A staff representative group is established to find the solution to workplace smoking issues. Through some funding allocation, the group is able put up 'no-smoking' signs and build a 'smoker's corner' outside the building. The group also organises sessions with staff about health consequences of smoking and provides resources about where to get help to quit.	To link new arrivals with employment opportunities, the group forms a partnership with two rural communities experiencing labour shortages. The group also ensures that these areas offer good access to housing and education, and a welcoming and supportive environment.	The LGA staff member works with a CALD* service provider and a local sports club to increase physical activity opportunities for CALD community members. The sports club builds capacity for adoption of healthy behaviours.

* Culturally and Linguistically Diverse

continued

165

Table 7.1 *continued*

Projects addressing	Smoking rates	Mental health and wellbeing	Physical activity levels
Organisational capacity	A workplace develops a policy to ban smoking inside and outside the building.	The partners support local schools to develop protocols and systems, and to access professional development to assist them in settling relocating children and their families.	The LGA reviews their governance structure and agrees that subcommittees would strengthen their internal decision-making processes.
System capacity	A government passing smokefree workplace legislation following strong lobbying by the community.	The project is evaluated to identify good practices and to determine the resources required to establish and maintain a relocation program. Findings will be used to plan future relocation programs and to advocate to government for sound policies and programs to support relocation.	The Municipal Public Health and Wellbeing Plan incorporates strategies and allocates resources to improve formal and informal physical activity opportunities for CALD communities.

Principles of capacity building

Arole and colleagues (2004) list five key principles for capacity building. In summary, these are:

1. Community members must be involved in planning, implementing and evaluating programs. The most vulnerable must also be involved in all elements of a program. Community capacity building is about working in partnership and supporting community decision making.

2. Improving community capacity increases health by empowering communities to address underlying causes of ill-health, such as lack of adequate nutrition, safe drinking water and clean environment.

3. Increased community capacity occurs through opportunities for increased networking and information exchange. Information sharing enhances community knowledge and methods of working together and allows community gaps to be identified and addressed.

4. Skill and knowledge transfer that supports capacity building is enhanced by relationships of mutual respect between the practitioner/program and the individual/community. One must respect the inherent capacity within all people and recognise that knowledge transfer is a two-way process.

5. Skills are best learned in practice, as distinct from the communication of a skill in an abstract conceptual way. Practice should be in the context of needs assessment, analysis of a situation, planning of a program and implementation of activities.

Hawe et al. (2001) developed a capacity building checklist from which objective scores of capacity can be determined within communities and gaps identified for further action. VicHealth (2003) expanded on these concepts to produce a number of capacity building checklists, along with other relevant information relating to this area in their online publication on measuring health promotion impacts (see www.health.vic.gov.au/healthpromotion).

WHO has also made a priority of building capacity for health promotion within its member countries in recent years. Its strategy is designed to integrate health promotion into the building blocks of financial and human resource planning, knowledge management and partnership building through fostering leadership capacity for health promotion. This stems from an understanding that countries differ widely in their capacity for health promotion and that this needs to be addressed in most developing countries in particular. Case study 7.1 describes the experience of WHO's Regional Office in the Western Pacific Region in developing health promotion leadership capacity at a country level.

Forming partnerships

Health promotion, perhaps more so than any other health discipline, cannot function in a vacuum. Capacity building incorporates advocacy and relies on having effective partnerships. Partnerships are an important vehicle for bringing together diverse skills and resources for more effective health promotion outcomes. Partnerships can increase the efficiency of systems that have an impact on health by making the best use of complementary resources.

CASE STUDY **7.1**

Health promotion leadership development program (ProLead)

In 2004, the WHO Western Pacific Region (WPRO) initiated a regional health promotion leadership development program, ProLead, to create a critical mass of leaders in health promotion to apply their knowledge and skills to local projects and conditions, but with a global mindset. ProLead recognised the real-life difficulties in bringing about systemic changes in policies, and aimed to provide inputs in transformative leadership and management abilities to in-country staff who are in actual or potential positions of leadership. The demand for ProLead grew and it was adapted and modified.

Significant infrastructural changes were seen in participating countries. In the Western Pacific Region, Malaysia, Mongolia, Tonga and the Republic of Korea have established health promotion foundations, and Lao PDR, Vietnam and Samoa are working towards setting up such infrastructure. Such foundations offer an innovative way of mobilising new resources for promoting health and can support research, innovation and the strengthening of health promotion capacities in the health sectors as well as in sectors such as education, sports, arts, environment and commerce.

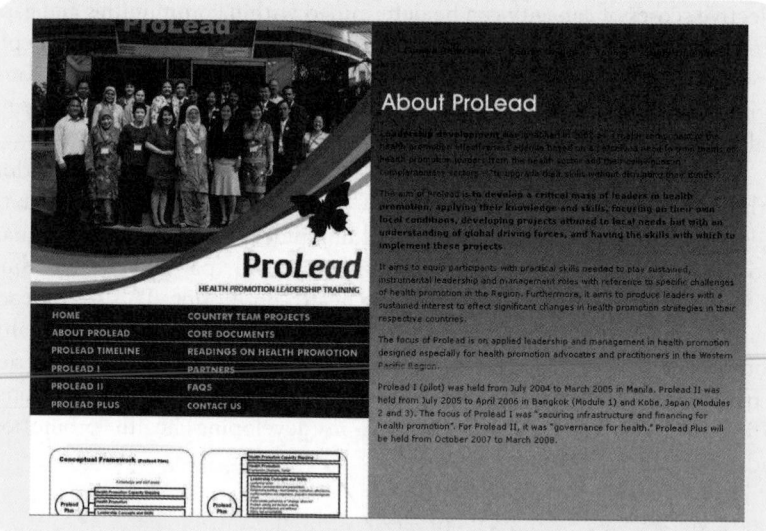

WHO 2009, www.who.int/healthpromotion, accessed May 2013

Interdisciplinary and intersectoral partnerships are needed at several different levels. Potential partners will be determined by the type of project in question. However these can include government departments, local government bodies, relevant non-government organisations (NGOs), community groups and academic and educational institutions. Although the selection of these may often seem obvious, a different perspective may need to be taken according to the diversity of the program. Reference materials are available for assisting health promotion practitioners to develop partnerships internationally (Pinet 2003), at the state level (Padget, Bekemeier & Berkowitz 2004) or for specific issues, such as heart disease (Nchiinda 2003).

VicHealth has developed a Partnerships Analysis Tool for developing and maintaining partnerships for health promotion. The aim of this tool is to help organisations reflect on the partnerships they have established and to monitor and maximise their effectiveness (VicHealth 2011).

Collaborative partnerships are a key component of community organisation and development processes and through their joint resourcing and planned action can make a potentially bigger impact on health outcomes across diverse sectors.

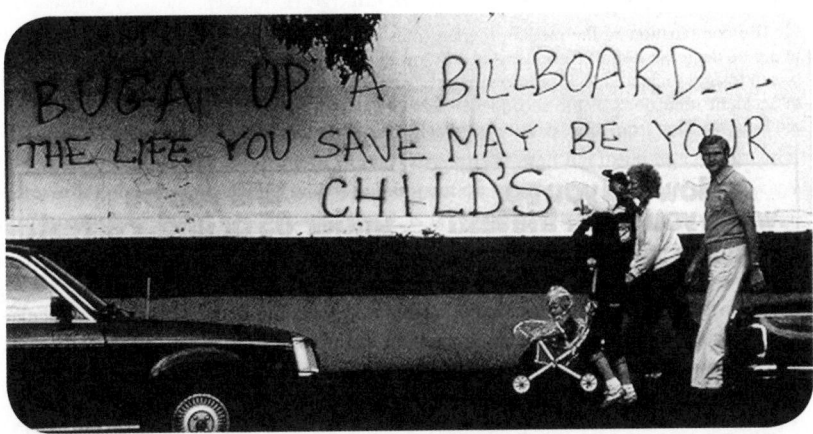

The work of BUGAUP (Billboard Utilising Graphitiists Against Unhealthy Promotions) to change the health environment in the 1980s

Community organisation and community development

As noted above, both community organisation and community development have a considerable intellectual history outside the public health area, particularly within social work, sociology, community welfare and community psychology. Where community organisation ends and community development begins is often a grey area. The essential difference between the two, however, is the relative proportion of decision making and control invested in the community. This is greater in community development than in community organisation.

Community organisation

Rothman (1968) defined three models of community organisation practice that remain valid today. These are social planning, social action and locality development.

Social planning emphasises a technical process of problem solving with regard to substantive social problems such as poverty, unemployment, inadequate housing, public transport and social isolation. It is an approach that attempts to solve community problems rationally within existing power structures. In this approach, community participation may vary from a great deal to a little—depending on the nature of the situation. The approach presupposes a level of technical knowledge and skills among planners who, it is assumed, can skilfully guide complex change processes.

Social action is an activist approach that attempts to shift power structures in a community through various methods of coercion or protest. It presupposes a generally disadvantaged or oppressed segment of the population that needs to be organised—perhaps in alliance with others—in order to make demands on the larger community for increased resources or treatment more in accordance with social justice principles. Examples are civil and worker rights, cause organisations and social movements where power structures or entrenched interests may be challenged.

Stages of social action

First they ignore you. Then they laugh at you. Then they fight you. Then you win.

—Mahatma Ghandi

Locality development aims to develop the potential of a community through self-help techniques and programs, within the constraints of the power structure. It rests on the assumption that community change may be pursued optimally through broad participation of a wide spectrum of people in goal determination and action at the local community level. Locality development is characterised by discussion and communication among a wide variety of different individuals, groups and factions, with the aim of achieving consensus. This construct from Rothman's (1968) typology most closely aligns with what is commonly referred to as community development. Examples include neighbourhood job skill development programs, community garden projects, migrant skill and esteem-building programs, and community literacy programs in adult education.

In reality, health promotion practitioners may need to draw on some combination of Rothman's three community organisation models. In some circumstances, the health issue may be significant enough to instigate a social movement for change.

The community organisation approach to health promotion has been most apparent in large-scale community intervention projects (with and without mass media support) designed to lower the risk of cardiovascular disease of populations such as in North Karelia, Finland (McAlister 1981); Stanford, California (Maccoby & Solomon 1981); Pawtucket, Rhode Island (Lasater, Carleton & LeFebvre 1988); the North Coast of New South Wales (Egger at al. 1983); and Wales (Nutbeam & Catford 1987).

Several reviews have been conducted in the decades since these large-scale health promotion interventions were conducted to reflect on their effectiveness. With regard to the Stanford Five-City Project, which began in 1978, numerous components of the intervention proved effective when evaluated individually, as was true in other community studies. However, the design limitations proved difficult to overcome, especially in the face of large, favourable risk factor changes in control sites. As a result, definitive conclusions about the overall effectiveness of the community-wide effects were not always possible. Nevertheless, in aggregate, these studies support the effectiveness of community-wide health promotion (Fortmann et al. 1995).

While the more behaviourally focused of these interventions showed little or no sustained impact, of all of them the North Karelia project, which began in Finland in 1972 in response to high cardiovascular disease (CVD) rates in that country in the late 1960s, was the most comprehensive and sustained. Using lifestyle modification methods and strategies for environmental change, major reductions were achieved in the three major risk factors: smoking rates, elevated blood cholesterol and blood pressure. Following on from the early success of the pilot project with significant reductions in the CVD risk factors, several major policy initiatives such as national tobacco legislation and nutrition policy were introduced in Finland as the project directly involved national health policy makers. Through coordinated health promotion action resourced at national and community level (see box on p. 172), the North Karelia project in Finland has shown the world that well-planned, theory-based and intensive community-based programs can be cost-effective and have a substantial impact on the lifestyle and risk factors of a population (Laatikainen, Vartiainen & Puska 2007).

National action in cardiovascular disease prevention in Finland

Major elements of Finnish national action in the national cardiovascular disease prevention program include the following:

1. Research and international research collaboration
2. Health services (especially primary health care)
3. North Karelia project and other demonstration programmes
4. Health promotion programmes (coalitions, NGOs, collaboration with media)
5. Schools, educational institutions
6. Collaboration with industry and business
7. Policy decisions, intersectoral collaboration, legislation
8. Health monitoring system: health behaviour, risk factors, nutrition, morbidity, mortality
9. International collaboration

Laatikainen, Vartiainen & Puska 2007

These large-scale public health programs have been comprehensive—that is, they have utilised a variety of different methods to achieve changes in individual behaviour and in community systems and structures and national health policy. An acceptance of the multifactorial nature of behaviour and environmental change has resulted in an eclectic framework for health promotion action that draws on a variety of different theoretical models.

Whereas most of the large public health interventions noted above were initiated by a central health authority or agency—making them closest to *social planning* of the three community organisation models in Rothman's (1968) typology—it can be seen that more 'from the ground up approaches' of information dissemination, behaviour change and maintenance of that change rely heavily on the involvement of community groups and organisations that could provide a vehicle for *locality* or *community development*.

The activities of community organisation in these programs have included training of community members so that they can contribute to creating a supportive environment for those making behavioural changes. The longer-term objective in targeting whole communities is to influence the climate of opinion on health issues in communities so that momentum can build for behavioural and structural changes to occur. Influence can occur directly by placing issues on the community agenda, and by creating interest and controversy through exposure to media messages and events. Influence can also occur indirectly by reaching the informal communication networks or channels that exist in peer groups, families and institutions.

Methods of community organisation

Methods of community organisation vary widely, but basically involve the following actions:

- *Determining the health needs of the community*—in respect of quantifiable or qualifiable factors. These may be related directly to health and determined from epidemiological statistics, or related indirectly, such as from community leaders' recommendations on the need for temporary accommodation for homeless youth. Methods include survey materials from the research literature, ad hoc surveys carried out by local government and other institutions, and formal and informal surveys and meetings with community opinion leaders.

- *Involving the community in planning*—the main vehicle of community involvement in community organisation has typically been the community or interest-group meeting, although the advent of electronic media has meant that this can also be used for real-time participation such as via Skype—particularly in remote areas. Both are aided by the processes of publicity media referred to in Chapter 5, as well as by direct invitation through interest groups. The latter is a more efficient technique because it is more personalised. Care should be taken to ensure that the organisation and running of planning functions is carried out democratically as it is likely that where both community members and technical experts are present, the tendency can be for the technical experts to dominate proceedings. However, in community organisation (compared with community development), the agenda is usually set and the meeting process must continually refer back to this agenda. If necessary, changes may be facilitated in the task process so that community involvement and ownership of the process is assured.

- *Facilitating action*—the process of organisation and planning should have, as its outcome, some form of action. This can include further mobilisation of resources, development of programs, involvement in individual or group activities and social action where necessary. Action, and the outcome of such action, should be the cornerstone of the community organisation process, informing the health promotion practitioner of the success of his/her intervention.

- *Changing health impacts and outcomes*—in the process of social and community organisation, it is often easy to overlook the original intent— which is to improve the health and/or and conditions of living that impact on health of the individual and the community in which such organisation is taking place. This may require quantitative follow-up measures (e.g. risk factor assessments) or qualitative assessments of quality of life. It may be worthwhile to note that subjective assessments of the value of any program tend to be tainted with personal biases (e.g. only positive responders respond) and, although it may be tempting to ascribe negative or zero effects to independent variables, the health professional should be resilient enough to prosper from accurate feedback.

CASE STUDY **7.2**

The Parents' Jury—a community advocacy program

The Parents' Jury, formed in 2004, is an online network of over 5500 parents, grandparents and guardians who are interested in improving the food and physical activity environments of Australian and New Zealand children. The jury's concerns include food marketing to kids, healthy schools, healthy checkouts, physical activity and healthy eating. As part of their community activism, the jury runs regular media events such as the annual 'Fame and Shame' awards, during which they nominate producers/marketers who have developed products that enhance or inhibit the health of children. They also run activist campaigns, stimulated by internet mailouts, aimed at advocating for change to improve child health. The jury has become an effective political lobby by targeting politicians through media releases and public relations activities.

For more detail see www.parentsjury.org.au.

Appropriate situations for community organisation

Community organisation is appropriate to most health promotion situations (Minkler 2004). Community organisation may link with individual, group and mass media methods where a strategy mix will require concurrent intervention at individual, group and population levels. In the case of the use of mass media, as noted previously, it is clearly indicated that media programs alone are not as effective as programs where media exposure is accompanied by community organisation (Flay 1987; Redman, Spencer & Sanson-Fisher 1990). These understandings have now led to health promotion program planners acknowledging the need to introduce community-based interventions in a strategy mix and not to rely on any single process.

The mass media alone will be unlikely to be effective unless system-level organisational, economic and environmental changes enable, and interpersonal communications reinforce, the behavioural change objectives.

CASE STUDY **7.3**

Building a healthy community at Mapoon, Cape York

The 'Planning for a Healthy Community Project' was funded by Queensland Health in 1995, with an explicit objective of improving environmental health outcomes. Two Indigenous people from Mapoon, a remote Indigenous community several hours drive from Weipa in Cape York, were employed as health promotion workers by Queensland Health and were instrumental in the project passing its initial approval stage. An interdisciplinary team of planners joined forces, including engineers, architects, landscape architects, technical trainers and appropriate technologists. The process was consistent with the traditions of action research, whereby a learning exchange was fostered between the local knowledge of the residents and the technical knowhow of the planners. The 'action' was the healthy community houses and infrastructure to come.

The project went to unusual lengths to follow a participatory process, including a household survey, interviews, focus groups, graphical imagery, design workshops and a project T-shirt. It included a planning committee and employment of a planning officer. Consultation proceeded beyond elected leaders and governing structures to Mapoon people at an individual and family level. It also included Mapoon people who were not living in Mapoon.

Early on the needs of Mapoon people were straightforward enough—the planners needed to recreate the spread-out layout of the original mission that had been the first settlement on the current site. A mining company had prospected the area, including aerial photography, at the height of the mission era prior to its closure and subsequent burning (and forced removal of its inhabitants) by the then Queensland Government in 1963. Aerial photography was five times magnified into a 6-metre strip. Taking this 'plan' back to Mapoon and laying it on the ground to people's animated excitement and drawing on transparent overlays became the landmark event of the project. Field teams walked through the bush with elders, locating old ruins, stumps and exotic fruit trees. Emergent global position system (GPS) technology digitally recorded locations that were then uploaded and mapped to a geographical information system (GIS).

Consistent with how the old mission had evolved, the housing plan as it developed was remarkably dispersed, in comparison to other communities of this nature: 95 per cent of people requested that houses be at least 50 metres apart, in comparison to the 10–20 metres typical to nearby Napranum community near Weipa. Each extended family block was to be one hectare, the equivalent of two football fields, surrounded by a perimeter bush buffer of a nominal 20 metres. Houses were architecturally designed to culturally appropriate layouts. Appropriate technology solutions were found, including rainwater tanks, onsite sewerage disposal and caravan-park style power outlets.

In 1995, a capital works program to the value of $3 million was awarded for Mapoon through two different infrastructure and housing programs. Mapoon was on the verge of an explosion of infrastructure on a scale that it had not previously seen. The planners were able to negotiate a high level of collaboration with the consulting engineers, construction supervisors and government officers that followed them. They brokered an unusual confluence of private and public sector operators—using the plan as a license for their action—as they tackled the many challenges of a dispersed settlement layout. Not only did the plan express the aspirations of Mapoon people, it also demonstrated the technical challenges had been thought through, sufficient for the engineers, project managers and government officials to pick up and run with.

Today, Mapoon still enjoys the same spread-out settlement layout. Many Mapoon people attribute the comparative lack of social problems in Mapoon to their houses not being crowded together like in other remote communities.

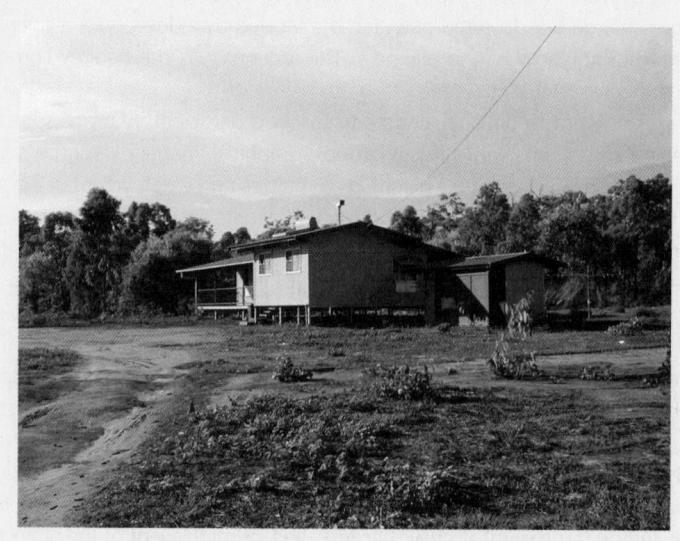

Old and new houses in Mapoon

Case study and photo courtesy of Professor Mark Moran, University of Queensland. See also Moran 1999.

Community development

Community development is the process of involving communities 'from the ground up' in their own decision making about factors related to health (Robinson & Green 2011). It concerns working with people and communities to develop their strength and confidence over an extended time period, as well as addressing immediate and pressing problems (Baum et al. 2012).

Until 1950, the community development process was generally characterised by government intervention or to overcome 'the inadequacies of colonial services in the fields of education, health and welfare' (Dixon 1989). Whereas self-help was stressed within the process, self-determination was not on the agenda, and community development, it appears, was wittingly and unwittingly used to create dependency on the sponsoring body—rather than independence from this body. Dixon (1989) commented on how community development had evolved at that time.

> In public policy terms, community development has, since the sixties, been a popular means of fostering participation in local-area service delivery, of obtaining the views and compliance of local leaders through consultation, and of encouraging self-help, volunteerism and cost-saving decentralisation. More recently, the securing of a sense of 'we-feeling' to counteract the problems of powerlessness and anomie, and to propel groups to collective action has been highlighted as valuable in the fields of local economic development, community mental health, adult education and social welfare.

Shabecoff and Brophy (2001) define community development as 'the economic, physical and social revitalisation of a community; led by the people who live in that community'. In this sense 'community developers do things with, not to or for, the community.'

Lin (1989) observed that, whereas community development in health promotion had previously been translated as 'the health promotion officer will do whatever the community wants him/her to do', there is now sufficient practice to develop a more rigorous approach to community development in health.

Given that such concepts are rarely static over time, community development has evolved and become aligned more recently with concepts of social capital. In fact Cox (1995) has described community development as a process of *developing* social capital. Social capital has several dimensions relevant to community development. These include building community connectedness and social inclusion, as well as achieving socio-political objectives such as influencing the allocation of resources to improve health for disadvantaged populations (Wakefield & Poland 2005).

At a grassroots level, service providers can enhance the social capital within a community by supporting community projects that bring neighbours together to achieve a mutually beneficial goal, such as beautifying the environment of a public housing estate, establishing a community fruit and vegetable garden or working with the local sporting club to encourage all parts of the community to participate in sporting activities (VicHealth 2011).

In health promotion, the community development perspective emphasises the importance of conceiving health promotion programs through a negotiated partnership with the communities whose cooperation and participation the health promotion practitioner seeks. A precondition for negotiations is an acceptance by the practitioner that the proposed program design may not be regarded as suitable by the communities to whom it is offered, or that management oversight might have to be shared or devolved. It should therefore be apparent that the brokering/negotiation/facilitation skills of the practitioner are key to effective community development approaches.

Applying community development

The nature of community development processes implies that they will be more effective among communities and sections of communities who are disempowered, where continuing inequalities exist with respect to health experience across class, gender, race and ethnicity, and where these groups are without the economic and social means to make decisions about their own lives (Jackson, Mitchell & Wright 1989). In Green and McAlister's terms, these are the 'hardest to reach' and are most likely to have the poorest health status. They are people who are:

> . . . typically disadvantaged in economic or status terms, they are socially more isolated or alienated, and they tend to be suspicious of organisations, including government agencies, purporting to help them. Their use of media is more exclusively for entertainment and their membership in organisations or coalitions is sporadic and limited to comparison with the early adopters. Reaching these people and organisations requires more expensive and labour-intensive forms of community organisation, communication and outreach. The payoff is often greater because of their high risk, but the cost per unit of service effectively delivered is necessarily higher (Green & McAlister 1984).

The community development approach, then, is most appropriate for, and can claim some successes in, lower socioeconomic and disadvantaged groups—such as in developing countries (Oakley 1989), among lower-income groups (El-Askari et al. 1998), and with Indigenous people (Copeman 2010). However, in some areas of concern—such as drug and alcohol abuse—community development approaches have been influential among all income groups (Reilly & Hommel 1988). These approaches have involved local schools, clubs, local governments and concerned citizens.

The role of the health promotion practitioner in the community development process is as a facilitator of action: to be as unobtrusive as possible, but to ensure that things happen. This role is not always an easy one and ethical dilemmas may arise for community organisers and developers—including health promotion practitioners—as they attempt to reconcile their mandate from both their employers and their communities—particularly if there are conflicting agendas (Minkler 1978). These realities are the reason for community developers not always being popular with everyone and sometimes even being regarded as 'ratbags'. However, Baum (1990) reminds us that the first medical officers of health appointed under the UK's Health of Towns movement in the nineteenth century could have been regarded as 'troublemakers' for health. In the context of the charter of the 'new' public health, Baum's call to action for practitioners in this field is still salient today. She suggests that:

> we must be prepared to be troublemakers for health—to rock the boat, to challenge the status quo and, perhaps most importantly, to question our own way of working and ensure our practice matches the rhetoric (Baum 1990).

In summary, community development in health should include the following elements:

- a thorough knowledge of the health and social problems of the area involved
- a thorough knowledge of the community itself—population, class, age structure, resources, power and influence groups, and knowledge of the usual processes of community action
- identification of leaders and influential people in the appropriate areas in the community—both elected and natural

CASE STUDY **7.4**

Big Brother Youth Mentoring Project for African–Australian Youth

The Awulian Community Development Association (AWCODA) Big Brother Youth Mentoring Project was introduced to build strength, skills and engagement among young African–Australians from the South Sudanese community who reside in South-east Queensland. South Sudanese young people are often left out of mainstream community development activities because of a lack of skills on their part and the wider community's reluctance to embrace different cultures. These young people face post-settlement challenges such as poor self-concept, social isolation, adverse home and life events, crowded rental households, disrupted pathways to employment and education, and socialising within limited networks. The AWCODA Big Brother Project began with a training program in focus group methodology for community elders. This methodology was then used to explore young people's perspectives on post-settlement issues and to develop a model for youth mentoring appropriate for their culture, values and practices. This led to a tailored mentoring program with elders, who could support those young people at risk of disengaging from work and/or education and whose needs are a priority not just for them but for the Awulian community.

Garang 2012; see also www.awcoda.com.au

- identification of natural neighbourhoods (see Kowachi & Berkman 2003)
- opinion surveys conducted in the community
- natural organisation of concerned groups and coalitions to consider identified problems
- emergence of representative planning groups to establish goals and plans for action
- development of neighbourhood committees
- training of volunteers if needed
- consistent feedback
- utilisation of available media
- maintained momentum.

Summary of community organisation and community development

Community organisation and community development differ in the degree of control and centralisation over program management that is held within the community itself. Community organisation principles are fundamental to most health promotion programs and can be an effective mechanism for gaining community involvement in programs that could be designed by a central body or health agency. Community development is most often appropriate in lower socioeconomic and disadvantaged neighbourhoods with underserved populations and for what have been sometimes described as settings with 'hard-to-reach' individuals and communities. Both systems have elements that are vital to the process of health promotion.

Particularly with reference to developing country contexts, and faced with new challenges from emerging diseases such as HIV/AIDS, natural disasters and the pressing need to improve standard of living in these countries, we find today that community-based approaches in health promotion are not 'out of fashion'. On the contrary, they are just as relevant as they ever were. Thanks to targeted investments in community-based projects made by agencies such as the World Bank, we now see international applications of these principles in the form of concepts such as *community mobilisation* being applied to health development. Community mobilisation embodies a demand-driven development approach whereby instead of decisions being made by experts, resources can be allocated based on the needs and preferences by the community itself and actions planned, carried out and evaluated by a community's individuals, groups and organisations on a participatory and sustained basis (World Bank 2011).

Career opportunities in health promotion

Health promotion work involving capacity building, community development and community organisation is usually part of a generalist health promotion practitioner's role. Work in this area as a health promotion speciality is available in developing countries through aid organisations and professional consulting organisations as well as with the World Health Organization. Local government and community-based organisations, such as youth and seniors organisations, require workers with these skills. Central and regional health agencies and primary healthcare organisations also employ health promotion officers specialising in community development and community organisation processes, particularly for rural and remote areas and in Indigenous communities. Community welfare and social workers are involved in capacity building through local and non-government organisations. Capacity-building skills are also sought after in private sector work for applications in coalition building, environmental and town planning and organisational development.

References

Arole, R., Fuller, B., & Deutschmann, P., 2004, Improving community capacity, in Moodie, R., & Hulme, A. (Eds), *Hands-on Health Promotion*, IP Communications, Melbourne.

Baum, F., 1990, Troublemakers for health, *In Touch* 7(1):5–6.

Baum, F., 2007, Cracking the nut of social equity: top down and bottom up pressure for action on the social determinants of health, *IUHPE—Promot Educ* 14(2):90–5.

Baum, F., Freeman, T., Lawless, A., & Jolley, G., 2012, Community development: improving patient safety by enhancing the use of health services, *Aust Fam Phys* 41(6):424–8.

Bracht, N.F., 1988, *Health Promotion at the Community Level: New Advances* (2nd edn), Sage Publications, Thousand Oaks, CA.

Brandstetter, S., McCool, M., Wise, M., & Loss, J., 2012, Australian health promotion practitioners' perceptions on evaluation of empowerment and participation, *Health Promot Int* 17 Sept [Epub ahead of print].

Brownell, K.D., 2004, *Food Fight*, Contemporary Books, New York.

Copeman., R.C., 2010, Assessment of Aboriginal health services, *Community Health Stud* 12(3):251–55.

Cox., E., 1995, *A Truly Civil Society*, ABC Books, Sydney.

Dixon., J., 1989, The limits and potential of community development for personal and social change, *Community Health Stud* 13(1):82–92.

Eade, D., 1997, *Capacity Building: An Approach to People-centred Development*, Oxfam, London.

Egger, G., Fitzgerald, W., Frape, G., Monaem, A., Rubinstein, P., Tyler, C., & Mackay, B., 1983, Results of a large-scale media anti-smoking campaign in Australia: the North Coast Healthy Lifestyle Programme, *BMJ* 287:1125–87.

Egger, G., Swinburn, B., & Islam, A., 2012, Economic growth and obesity: an interesting relationship with world-wide implications, *Econ Human Biol* 10(2):147–53.

El-Askari, G., Freestone, J., Irizarry, C., Kraut K.L., Mashiyama, S.T., Morgan, M.A., & Walton, S., 1998, The Healthy Neighbourhoods Project: a local health department's role in catalyzing community development, *Health Educ Behav* 25(2):146–59.

Flay, B.R., 1987, Mass media and smoking cessation: a critical review, *Am J Public Health* 77(2):153–60.

Fortmann, S.P., Flora, J.A., Winkleby, M.A., Schooler, C., Taylor, C.B., & Farquhar, J., 1995, Community intervention trials: reflections on the Stanford Five-City Project Experience, *Am J Epidemiol* 142(6): 576–86.

Garang, P.M., 2012, *AWCODA Guide for African-Australian Youth Mentoring*, Awulian Community Development Association, Toowoomba, available at www.awcoda.com.au.

Green, L.W., & McAlister, A.L., 1984, Macro-intervention to support health behaviour: some theoretical perspectives and practical reflections, *Health Educ Quart*erly 11(3):332–9.

Hawe, P., King, L., Noort, M., Jornens, C., & Lloyd, B., 2001, *Indicators to Help with Capacity Building in Health Promotion*, Australian Centre for Health Promotion, NSW Health.

Jackson, T., Mitchell, S., & Wright, M., 1989, The community development continuum, *Community Health Stud* 13(1):66–73.

Katz, R., 1984, *Empowerment and Synergy: Expanding the Community's Healing Resources, Studies in Empowerment*, The Haworth Press, New York.

Kersh,R. & Morone, J., 2002, The politics of obesity: seven steps to government action, *Health Aff* (Millowood), 21(6):142–53.

Kowachi, I., & Berkman, L.F., (Eds), 2003, *Neighbourhoods and Health*, Oxford University Press, Oxford.

Laatikainen, T., Vartiainen, E., & Puska, P., 2007, The North Karelia lessons for prevention of cardiovascular disease, *Italian J Public Health* 4(2):97–101.

Lasater, T.M., Carleton, R.A., & LeFebvre, R.C., 1988, The Pawtucket Heart Health Programme: utilizing community resources for primary prevention, *Rhode Island Med J* 71:63–7.

Lin, V., 1989, Education, prevention and social realities, Paper presented at the Fourth National Drug Educator's Workshop, Adelaide.

Maccoby, N., & Solomon, D.S., 1981, The Stanford Community Studies in Heart Disease Prevention, in Rice, R.E. & Paisley, W.J. (Eds), *Public Communication Campaigns*, Sage Publications, Thousand Oaks, CA.

Mackenbach, J.P., 2012, The persistence of health inequalities in modern welfare states: the explanation of a paradox, *Soc Sci Med* 75(4):761–9.

Marmot, M.G., 1999, *Social Determinants of Health*, Oxford University Press, London.

McAlister, A., 1981, Anti-smoking campaigns: progress in developing effective communications, in Rice, R.E. & Paisley, W.J. (Eds), *Public Communication Campaigns*, Sage Publications, Thousand Oaks, CA.

Minkler, M., 1978, Ethical issues in community organization, *Health Educ Monographs* Summer:198–210.

Minkler, M. (Ed), 2004, *Community Organizing and Community Building for Health*, Rutger's University Press, New Jersey.

Moran, M., 1999, *Improved settlement planning and environmental health in remote Aboriginal communities*, Report no. cat 99/6, Centre for Appropriate Technology, available at www.planning.org.au/documents/item/2542.

Nchiinda, T.C., 2003, Research capacity development for CVD prevention: the role of partnerships, *Ethn Dis* 13(2 Suppl 2):540–4.

Nutbeam, D., & Catford, J., 1987, The Welsh Heart Program evaluation strategy: progress, plans and possibilities, *Health Promot* 2(1):5–18.

Oakley, P., 1989, *Community Involvement in Health Development: an Examination of the Critical Issues*, World Health Organization, Geneva.

O'Dowd, A., 2012, Fight to tackle unhealthy lifestyles has widened gap in health inequalities, *BMJ* 345:e5707.

Offer, A., Pechy, R., & Ulijaszek, S., 2010, Obesity under affluence varies by welfare regimes: the effect of fast food, insecurity, insecurity and inequality, *Econ Human Biol* 8:297–308.

Padget, S.M., Bekemeier, B., & Berkowitz, B., 2004, Collaborative partnerships at the state level; promoting systems changes in public health infrastructure, *J Pub Health Manag Pract* 10(3):251–7.

Pinet, G., 2003, Global partnerships: a key challenge and opportunity for implementation of international health law, *Med Law* 22(4):561–77.

Redman, S., Spencer, E., & Sanson-Fisher, R., 1990, The role of the mass media in changing health related behaviour: a critical appraisal of two models, *Health Promot Int* 5(1):85–101.

Reilly, C., & Hommel, P., 1988, *Strategies for the Prevention of Drug and Alcohol Problems*, Directorate of the Drug Offensive, New South Wales Department of Health, Sydney.

Robinson, J.W., & Green, G.P., 2011, *Introduction to Community Development: Theory, Practice and Service-learning*, Sage Publications, New York.

Rothman, J., 1968, *Three Models of Community Organisation Practice*, National Conference on Social Welfare, Social Work Practice, Columbia University Press, New York.

Shabecoff, A., & Brophy, C., 2001, *A Guide to Careers in Community Development*, Island Press, Washington DC.

Stringhini, S., Berkman, L., Dugravot, A., Ferrie, J.E., Marmot, M., Kivimaki, M., & Singh-Manoux, A., 2012, Socioeconomic status, structural and functional measures of social support, and mortality: the British Whitehall II Cohort Study, 1985–2009, *Am J Epidemiol* 15;175(12):1275–83.

Syme, L.S., 2003, Social determinants of health: the community as empowered partner, Paper presented to the Communities in Control Conference (convened by Community and Catholic Social Services), Melbourne, April.

Thompson, B., & Kinne, S., 1990, Social change theory: applications to community health, in Bracht, N. (Ed.), *Health Promotion at the Community Level*, Sage Publications, Thousand Oaks, CA, pp. 45–65.

Tsey, K., Whiteside, M., Haswell-Elkins, M., Bainbridge, R., Cadet-James, Y., & Wilson, A., 2010, Empowerment and Indigenous Australian Health: a synthesis of findings from Family Wellbeing formative research, *Health and Health Care in the Community* 18(2): 169–79.

Van Daele, T., Van Audenhove, C., Hermans, D., Van Den Bergh, O., & Van Den Brouke, S., 2012, Empowerment implementation: enhancing fidelity and adaptation in a psycho-education intervention, *Health Promot Int* 19 Dec [Epub ahead of print].

VicHealth, 2003, *Measuring Health Promotion Impacts: A Guide to Impact Evaluation in Integrated Health Promotion*, Victorian Government Department of Human Services, Melbourne.

VicHealth, 2011, *The Partnerships Analysis Tool*, Victorian Health Promotion Foundation, Melbourne, available at www.health.vic.gov.au/healthpromotion.

Wakefield, S.E.L., & Poland, B., 2005, Family, friend or foe? Critical reflections on the relevance and role of social capital in health promotion and community development, *Soc Sci Med* 60: 2819–32.

Wakefield, M.A., & Wilson, D.A., 1985, Community organisation for health promotion, *Community Health Stud* 10(4):444–50.

Wallerstein, N., 1992, Powerlessness, empowerment and health: implications for health promotion programs, *Am J Health Promot* 6(3):197–205.

Wallerstein, N., 2002, Empowerment to reduce health disparities, *Scand J Public Health* (Suppl) 59:72–7.

Wallerstein, N., 2006, *What Is the Evidence on Effectiveness of Empowerment to Improve Health?* WHO Regional Office for Europe (Health Evidence Network report), Copenhagen, available at www.euro.who.int/Document/E88086.pdf.

Weatherburn, C. 2012, Health inequalities in primary care: time to face justice, *Brit J Gen Pract* 62(603):517.

World Bank, 2011, *Participatory Planning and Community Mobilization*, Washington, DC, available at www.worldbank.org.

WHO (World Health Organization), 1986, *Ottawa Charter for Health Promotion*, International Conference on Health Promotion, Ottawa, 21 November.

WHO, 1999, *The World Health Report 1999: Making a Difference*, WHO, Geneva.

Wilkinson, R., & Pickett, K., 2010, *The Spirit Level: Why Greater Equality Makes Societies Stronger*, Bloomsbury Press, New York.

chapter **8**

Focus on populations: environmental approaches

Summary of main points

- By making the healthy choice an easier choice (and sometimes the only choice), environmental approaches can be more effective than trying to change behaviours to achieve better health.
- Environments can be thought of as physical, economic, socio-cultural or political.
- Environmental interventions include policy, regulation and legislation, technological changes, organisational interventions and the use of incentives and disincentives.
- Technological change, such as the use of sunscreens for skin cancer, represents a means to harness innovation for health advancement.
- The ANGELO process is one way of diagnosing unhealthy environments.
- Economic and political considerations weigh heavily on environmental issues.
- Without economic and environmental attention, health promotion needs to adopt an 'environmental lens' as the potential population-level gains afforded by health promotion efforts could be compromised by environmental degradation, which would be like 'cooking dinner while the house is burning' (Dunnette 1989).

The value of health-promoting policy

The perennial question in health promotion is 'Which strategy is most effective?'. As noted previously, this book does not come down on the side of any single strategy or approach. We present the philosophy that selecting from a health promotion toolkit with a range of different strategies and methods available and appropriate to each context, often applied in combination, is likely to be the most effective approach in dealing with contemporary health issues and problems.

However, if one approach *were* to be favoured above others, the scales of evidence weigh most heavily in favour of population-level policies that modify the health environment in all its dimensions and do not rely solely on individuals changing unhealthy behaviours. This approach is about changing the environmental context to make individuals' 'default decisions' healthy ones. For example, Pearson (2011) cites evidence to demonstrate that public policy interventions in the second half of the twentieth century have led to changes in the physical, economic and social context that have significantly reduced population risk and death rates from heart disease and stroke in the US and elsewhere.

As well as the (often considerable) time it can take for the health promotion practitioner to influence the policy-making process, perhaps the bigger question and potential obstacle to change is the degree to which any community will accept or support policy changes that may impact on an individual's perceived rights to exercise free choice, despite the health benefits that may accrue from the proposed policy. This will vary from community to community, from nation to nation and over time. Healthy public policy gains are generally hard won against opposition: for philosophical reasons, for commercial reasons, because people do not understand the evidence and simply because of resistance to change. For example, Professor Mike Daube recently reminded us that back in 1851, when the UK was moving towards its great sanitary revolution led by the pioneering epidemiologist, John Snow, an editorial in the *London Times* thundered, 'We prefer to take our chances of cholera and the rest than be bullied by Mr Snow. Every man is entitled to his own dungheap!' (Daube 2012).

Modifying the environment

The strategies and methods dealt with so far in this book involve direct interventions with individuals, groups or whole populations—often focusing on intrapersonal and interpersonal factors. More indirect means of influencing a population's health include 'passively' changing environments that encourage ill-health by manipulating the environment or developing public policy for health benefit, for example, by introducing regulations and legislation, introducing organisational and other settings-based adaptations, and applying incentives and disincentives. Robinson and Sirard (2005) refer to passive changes that have active benefits as 'stealth' interventions: those that are done for another purpose but have a side effect of inadvertently promoting health. Egger (2007) identifies carbon trading initiatives, intended to affect carbon emissions and climate change, as an example of a stealth intervention, since they could also help reduce obesity by encouraging greater use of person-power (e.g. walking/cycling) and less use of non-renewable resources (e.g. petrol, fatty processed foods).

The importance of creating supportive environments achieved formal recognition with the Ottawa Charter in 1986. Since then, more specific environmental models have been developed for dealing with a variety of contemporary health issues (Egger & Swinburn 1997, 2013; Swinburn, Egger & Raza 1999). Environments in this context should not be considered as only physical. They include economic, political or socio-cultural environments. In addition, there are micro-environments, or those in immediate proximity to the target population, sometimes considered as 'settings'; and macro-environments, or those encompassing industry, economic and employment groups, considered as 'sectors'.

As Simmons and colleagues (2009) have observed in relation to obesity, the social, political and economic environment may encourage or reinforce health-damaging behaviours and may discourage people even from desiring to engage in healthy behaviours. Advertisements for high-fat foods, cigarettes and alcoholic drinks often create a social environment, particularly among sub-groups such as teenagers, who may be more susceptible to appeals that make smoking or drinking look like the road to success and popularity. The environment may also discourage people from engaging in health-enhancing actions—even when they want to do so—by providing obstacles like high prices, lack of availability and social stigma to such behaviour.

Health-promoting policies can modify social, political and economic influences. For example, to discourage smoking, especially among adolescents, health promotion advocates have successfully lobbied for increased taxes on tobacco products—especially to discourage the uptake of smoking (Bierer & Rigotti 1992). Environmental measures have the advantage of cost-effectiveness, influencing population groups that are often hard to reach, and having a more lasting effect on behaviour change because they become incorporated into structures, systems, policies and socio-cultural norms (Swinburn, Egger & Raza 1999).

The approaches that can be considered under the strategy of *environmental adaptations* are:

- physical modifications to the environment
- physical and social regulation and legislation
- technological interventions
- organisational interventions
- the use of incentives and disincentives.

Advocacy for change could also be considered in this category, but because this has been considered in Chapter 6, it will not be discussed again here.

CASE STUDY **8.1**

The influence of changes in the environment over time

Some novel Australian research shows how small, subtle changes in the environment can mount up to have a large, long-term influence on health. A group of actors who play the part of soldiers, convicts and settlers at Old Sydney Town, a theme park north of Sydney in New South Wales, were asked to live in for a week and not use modern technology at all during that time, while wearing special movement sensors to detect activity levels. Results were then compared with that of a group of sedentary urban office workers in modern-day Sydney. The average difference amounted to around 1000 kilocalories of energy per day, or the equivalent of walking approximately 16 kilometres more in the early nineteenth century than in the early twenty-first century.

A theoretical postulation of changes in activity levels is shown in Figure 8.1.

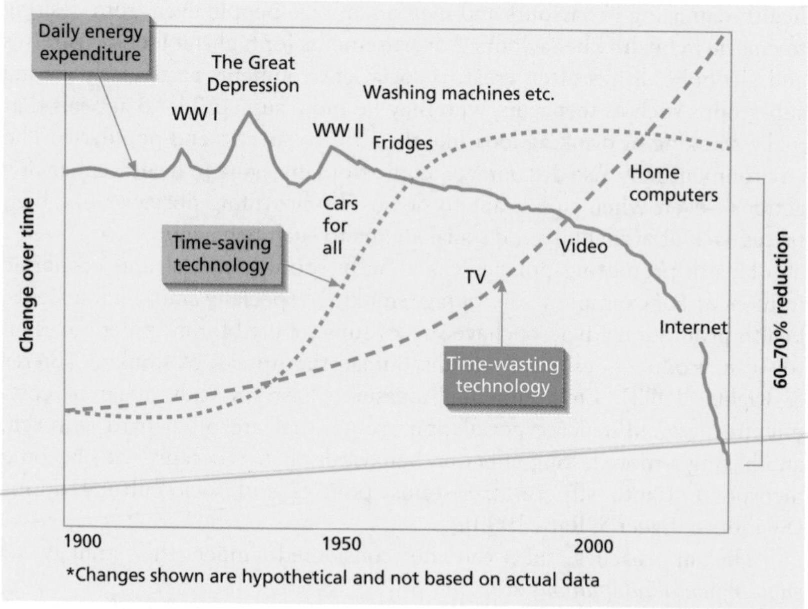

*Changes shown are hypothetical and not based on actual data

Figure 8.1: Postulated changes in physical activity levels over time with changes in technology

Vogels et al. 2004

This suggests that while activity levels in the general population would have been expected to increase during the Great Depression and both world wars, big decreases probably coincided with the introduction of 'time-saving' technology (e.g. cars, refrigerators, washing machines) after the 1950s. This was added to by the development of 'time-using' technology (e.g. videos, electronic games,

TV), and more recently by the significant effects of personal electronic devices (e.g. laptops, iPads, smartphones) and the internet. Such declines show the power of the environment in affecting modern health, and are likely to have significantly contributed to the modern obesity epidemic.

Vogels et al. 2004

Behaviour of a long-standing nature—such as diet or exercise—is notoriously difficult to change. Changes to the physical environment, which deliver positive health benefits, can sometimes be made relatively easily. For example, traffic accident research shows that the fatality rate from motor vehicles is significantly decreased when the structure of highways is changed (Wu 2012). Another example is in the provision of bike/pedestrian pathways where these can facilitate active transport, saving carbon fuel resources and increasing physical activity. Economic benefits can also accrue. For example, a cost–benefit analysis conducted by Wang and colleagues (2005) in Nebraska, US, found that every dollar invested in these pathways produced a return of almost three dollars in reduced medical costs.

A further example of health-related environmental change comes from the area of nutrition. It is now well accepted that a lowering of total fat in the diet is a vital aspect of improving the health of the population. However, because high-fat foods are readily available, tasty and cheap, it is difficult to influence behaviour in a positive direction. In New Zealand, a survey of fast food outlets showed that the average fat content of hot chips (French fries) was 11.5 per cent. Researchers showed that this was able to be reduced by 1.5 per cent by simple changes in cooking practices, which would then result in an estimated decrease in per capita fat consumption of 0.5 kilogram per year and hence a significant decrease in unhealthy body weight of the average New Zealander (Morley-John et al. 2002).

Changing nutrition policy at a national level can have even more dramatic consequences for health improvement. For example, Poland discontinued price supports for butter and high-fat meats and allowed the importation of fruits, vegetables and low saturated fat margarines after the break-up of the former Soviet Union in the early 1990s. This was followed by a rapid 26 per cent decrease in coronary disease mortality in that country (Zatonski & Willet 2005).

Injury is another area that is particularly influenced by environmental change. Injury is the third-largest cause of death (after heart disease and cancers) in Australia and New Zealand, but is responsible for many more years of potential life lost—because it is the most common cause of death in people aged under 40 years. US engineer Dr William Haddon led a paradigm shift in thinking in this area in 1974 when he redefined traffic injury in epidemiological terms and showed that the appropriate intervention for injury prevention

CASE STUDY **8.2**

Changing ships for better health

The influence of subtle changes in the environment on health is exemplified by a US Navy study comparing surreptitious changes to a low diet in one US Navy ship compared to a second ship where no such change occurred over a 6-month deployment. Cooks on the test ship (Ship A) were instructed on cooking to American Cardiology Society guidelines. Exercise was also encouraged in the test ship, but shops, vending machines and other factors remained unchanged. Standard navy menus were unchanged on the control ship (Ship B).

Results after 6 months are shown in the table below, suggesting a major impact of a subtle change in ship A's environment.

	Ship A	Ship B
Mean weight change	−5.3 kg	+3.1 kg
Mean waist change	−4.8 cm	+3.6 cm
In those greater than 90 kg at start	74% lost weight 26% gained weight	26% lost weight 74% gained weight

Swinburn 2002

is relatively easy, requiring only simple modifications to the environment (although these modifications must be accompanied by a shift in community attitude to the view that 'injuries *are* preventable') (Haddon 1980).

Successes in injury prevention through environmental modifications include:

- a 50 per cent reduction in the frequency and severity of belted passengers in newer, compared to older, cars in France (Page et al. 2012)
- a reduction in injuries in the home due to home safety education and provision of safety equipment (Kendrick et al. 2012)
- a 73 per cent reduction in swimming pool drownings in children through erection of proper barriers around home pools (Thompson & Rivara 2003)
- a 50 per cent decrease in concussions and an 80 per cent reduction in skull fractures in bike riders aged under 14 years wearing helmets (Bergenstal et al. 2012).

The lesson from these examples provides further evidence that if there are choices of strategy, a first priority should be to seek to alter the environment before tackling more difficult behavioural or social changes

(Mock et al. 2004). The National Injury Surveillance Unit was established as a federal initiative to monitor causes of and changes in injuries throughout Australia, and is now a part of the Australian Institute for Health and Welfare, operating as a research centre of Flinders University (see www.nisu.flinders.edu.au). State health and transport departments have also taken on the area of injury prevention and some states have bodies such for reducing specific injuries such as through motor vehicle accidents.

Health in All Policies

Building healthy public policy remains one of the five areas listed for action in the Ottawa Charter for Health Promotion (WHO 1986). This means that in all sections and at all levels of government (including local, regional and national levels), policy makers must be aware of, and accept responsibility for, the health consequences of their decisions.

While this action area is still a valid goal for health promotion today, it is nevertheless difficult to implement at the level where macro-level health policy decisions are made. The reality for contemporary health departments and central agencies is that functions relating to building regulatory policies have largely become the domain of other agencies to administer. As a consequence, the focus within health departments on the regulatory role has diminished, displaced by a focus on (clinical) health services and related programs (Penman 2008). Meanwhile other government departments such as environmental protection, primary industries and agriculture, transport, and workplace health and safety carry most of the regulatory responsibilities that directly impact on the health of populations.

This relative interdependence of public policy around health has led to calls for a new approach to governance in this area in the form of more 'joined-up' government action, which would see the development of strategic plans that set out common goals, integrated responses and increased accountability across government departments. This clearly also requires the involvement of community groups and the private sector. This approach, led by the World Health Organization (WHO), is referred to as 'Health in All Policies' and has been developed and tested in a number of countries. It assists leaders and policy makers to integrate considerations of health, wellbeing and equity during the development, implementation and evaluation of policies and services (WHO 2010). Some examples of 'joined-up' government action across a range of sectors and issues from the 2010 *Adelaide Statement on Health in All Policies* can be found in Table 8.1.

Table 8.1: **Examples of 'joined-up' government action**

Sectors and issues	Interrelationships between health and wellbeing
Economy and employment	• Economic resilience and growth is stimulated by a healthy population. Healthier people can increase their household savings, are more productive at work, can adapt more easily to work changes and can remain working for longer. • Work and stable employment opportunities improve health for all people across different social groups.
Security and justice	• Rates of violence, ill-health and injury increase in populations whose access to food, water, housing, work opportunities and a fair justice system is poorer. As a result, justice systems within societies have to deal with the consequences of poor access to these basic needs. • The prevalence of mental illness (and associated drug and alcohol problems) is associated with violence, crime and imprisonment.
Education and early life	• Poor health of children or family members impedes educational attainment, reducing educational potential and abilities to solve life challenges and pursue opportunities in life. • Educational attainment for both women and men directly contributes to better health and the ability to participate fully in a productive society, and creates engaged citizens.
Agriculture and food	• Food security and safety are enhanced by consideration of health in food production, manufacturing, marketing and distribution through promoting consumer confidence and ensuring more sustainable agricultural practices. • Healthy food is critical to people's health, and good food and security practices help to reduce animal-to-human disease transmission, and are supportive of farming practices with positive impacts on the health of farm workers and rural communities.
Infrastructure, planning and transport	• Optimal planning for roads, transport and housing requires the consideration of health impacts as this can reduce environmentally costly emissions, and improve the capacity of transport networks and their efficiency with moving people, goods and services. • Better transport opportunities, including cycling and walking opportunities, build safer and more liveable communities, and reduce environmental degradation, enhancing health.

Environments and sustainability	• Optimising the use of natural resources and promoting sustainability can be best achieved through policies that influence population consumption patterns, which can also enhance human health. • Globally, a quarter of all preventable illnesses are the result of the environmental conditions in which people live.
Housing and community services	• Housing design and infrastructure planning that take account of health and wellbeing (e.g. insulation, ventilation, public spaces, refuse removal) and involve the community can improve social cohesion and support for development projects. • Well-designed, accessible housing and adequate community services address some of the most fundamental determinants of health for disadvantaged individuals and communities.
Land and culture	• Improved access to land can support improvements in health and wellbeing for Indigenous peoples as Indigenous peoples' health and wellbeing are spiritually and culturally bound to a profound sense of belonging to land and country. • Improvements in Indigenous health can strengthen communities and cultural identity, improve citizen participation and support the maintenance of biodiversity.

Government of South Australia, 2010, *Adelaide Statement of Health in All Policies*, WHO, Geneva.

Industry policy changes required for obesity control in children

Food sales and marketing have become a major concern in light of big increases in obesity in school-age children around the world. In a comprehensive analysis of approaches to deal with this, US obesity expert, Dr Kelly Brownell has suggested that:

> the time has come for the (food and soft drink) industry to determine that it will be a trustworthy public health ally by adopting the following practices: (1) suspend all food advertising and marketing campaigns directed at children; (2) remove sugar-sweetened soft drinks and snack foods from vending machines in schools; (3) end sponsorship of scholastic activities and professional nutrition organizations linked to product promotion; and (4) refrain from political contributions that might influence national nutritional policy.

Calls for private corporations to show restraint in advertising and promotion of commercial products that are potentially damaging are ongoing. Health officials need to be eternally vigilant as the profit motive makes unregulated industry an unlikely respecter of social wellbeing. The rise of high caffeine 'energy' drinks, and their potential overuse by susceptible youth (Sepkowitz 2013), and increased injury risk when mixed with alcohol (Howland & Rohsenhow 2013) is a case in point.

Brownell 2004

CASE STUDY **8.3**

ANGELO: a diagnostic tool for identifying unhealthy environments

ANGELO, an ANalysis Grid for Environments Leading to Obesity, was developed initially to help communities diagnose aspects of their environment that may enhance or discourage obesity and identify potential interventions. The grid consists of four environmental types and two sizes (see text for a discussion of these) defining settings and sectors in a community.

The questions shown in the grid are put to stakeholders to identify key obesogenic elements and these are then ranked according to local relevance, potential impact and changeability, to identify high-priority areas for intervention.

A grid for diagnosing environments

Environment type/size	Micro-environment (settings)		Macro-environment (sectors)	
	Food	Physical activity	Food	Physical activity
Physical	[What is available?]			
Economic	[What are the financial factors?]			
Policy	[What are the rules?]			
Socio-cultural	[What are the attitudes, beliefs, perceptions and values?]			

The grid has been used in stakeholder groups in several Pacific Island communities to encourage community participation and focus actions for 'diabesity' prevention. After getting stakeholders to fill in the matrix by brainstorming environmental issues, the grid is then 'lifted' and choices ranked with consideration of possible solutions.

The ANGELO approach is a facilitatory tool, which enables community members to recognise causal issues that may otherwise be less clear. Examples from the Pacific include roaming dogs that stop islanders walking (physical environment), attitudes to women exercising in public and during pregnancy (socio-cultural), cost and availability of low-fat fresh food (economic) and excessive TV watching among children (changes in family activities).

ANGELO is not meant to provide answers to environmental issues. These should come from the community itself. It does, however, provide an enlightened perspective and community involvement in ongoing interventions.

Egger, Swinburn & Rossner 2002

Regulation and legislation

In some circumstances, legislation (by making the healthy choice the *only* choice), backed up by enforcement, can be the only effective way of ensuring healthy behaviour where compliance must be guaranteed for public health and/or safety. Measures such as the compulsory wearing of seatbelts, setting blood alcohol limits and doing random breath testing have resulted in a decrease in road traffic accidents in most areas where they have been introduced. In Australia, these measures were effective only when they were backed up by enforcement measures (for example, see Figure 8.2).

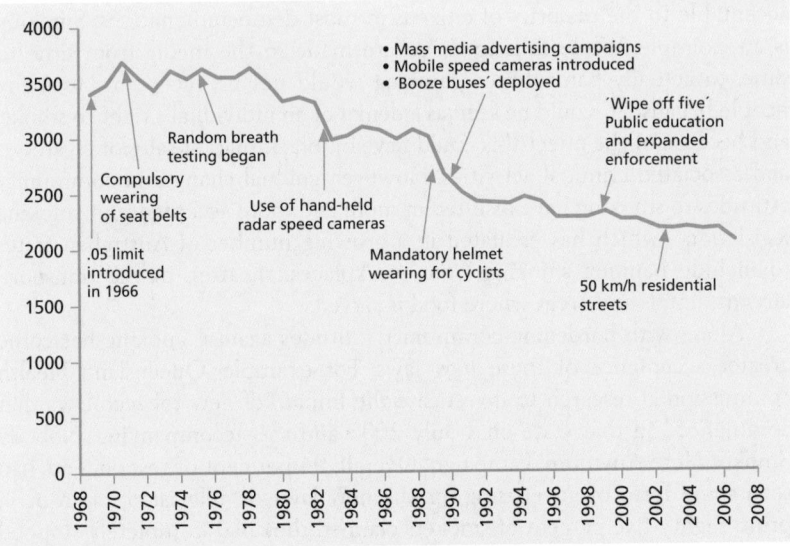

Figure 8.2: Road fatalities in Australia 1968–2008
NPHT 2009, Transport Accident Commission of Victoria

The significant difference in traffic-accident injury rates between Australia and the US has been attributed to the early introduction of compulsory seatbelt use and drink-driver restrictions in Australia. Differences in homicide rates between the two countries have similarly been put down to firearm-enforcement laws in Australia (Sleet 1990).

Another example, no less important to public health, particularly in countries of the tropical world including developed nations such as Singapore, relates to dengue fever control. Despite appeals to householders via health promotion campaigns for them to throw out containers such as buckets and tyres that can hold stagnant water, authorities in these countries have found these campaigns have been only partially effective in preventing dengue outbreaks. As a dengue fever epidemic can be sustained with a relatively small number of breeding containers in any locality once the dengue virus is transmitted from an infected person to mosquitoes that carry it (these mosquitoes breed in mostly artificial containers carrying stagnant water lying around the home and yard), governments have passed laws and resorted to inspecting premises and imposing heavy fines where

195

mosquito-breeding containers are found. In this case enforcement is a last resort but possibly a necessary one when the placed against the huge potential human health and economic consequences of allowing large dengue outbreaks to occur unchecked (see Ooi, Kee-Tai & Gubler 2006).

Legislative controls and restrictions over health-compromising behaviours, without going to the point of making them illegal, may be more acceptable to the majority of citizens in most democratic nations. Smoking is an example. While calls to do so are made in the media from time to time, to actually ban tobacco smoking would not be acceptable to many people because it would be seen as a denial of an individual's right to smoke, and because of the effect this could have on black-market sales of cigarettes and associated criminal activities. However, gradual changes in community attitudes to smoking have resulted in more and more acceptance of smoking legislation—which has escalated in a growing number of Australian states to include banning smoking from workplaces, theatres, public transport, aircraft, hotels and areas where food is served.

Along with hardening community attitudes against smoking has come greater acceptance of these new laws. For example, Queensland Health commissioned research to investigate the impact of new tobacco laws that commenced in that state on 1 July 2006 and the accompanying 'Nobody Smokes Here Anymore' campaign. Overall, 94 per cent of respondents had seen some form of advertising for the new laws on television, radio or in print. Eighty-five percent of smokers claimed they had 'completely stopped smoking in all areas where it is illegal to smoke at all times' and two-thirds (67%) reported 'smoking less in public spaces' generally (IUATLD 2007).

Nevertheless, a considered analysis of improvements in smoking rates has shown that while improvements have been considerable, these could be much greater with more committed government support. While just $176 million was spent on tobacco control in Australia from 1970–1998, the net revenue accruing to government from tobacco taxes (sometimes referred to as 'sin taxes') in the same time period was $8.4 billion (Chapman 2004).

Introducing new legislation can be a long-term process. Because the health promotion practitioner often works within defined parameters, the power of one person or even one organisation to influence legislative change is limited (although not impossible). Health promotion practitioners may need to utilise some of the strategies of community organisation suggested in Chapter 7 to mobilise public support and/or acceptance of new legislation.

The great 'nanny state' debate

Whenever a new law or government policy is mooted or its introduction is pending, the media often 'lights up' with claims that this represents a further example of the government interfering in the private lives of its citizens and rapidly becoming a 'nanny state'! The release of a number of recommendations of the Australian Government's National Preventative Health Taskforce in 2009 caused just such a response in the Australian media. Professor Leonie Segal, prominent health economist and academic, weighed into the debate, providing some more rational perspectives. Following are some comments taken from an article at the time:

> When governments introduce regulation to control food quality or unsafe work practices or create national parks, we rarely hear the cry 'nanny state'. But when it comes to promoting health and well-being, by seeking to discourage harmful health lifestyle behaviours, the cry 'nanny state' is heard, from some Members of Parliament, policy 'think tanks', and others. It is readily apparent that health and health care and the adoption of lifestyle behaviours do not approximate the 'perfect market'. Not only are citizens provided with incomplete information about food and alcohol and the health consequences, they also face a barrage of persuasive advertising, designed to influence their choices, not inform. In short, in relation to lifestyle behaviours, the unfettered market will not maximise social gain. This provides a clear rationale for government to intervene. It is not about 'dictating how we lead our lives'; it is about addressing distorted incentives that undermine the total societal health and well-being. The question is not whether or not distortions should be addressed by government: that is clear if maximising well-being is the societal goal. The only real question is how this should be done. Efficiency is the core logic underpinning the need for a government preventive strategy. But of course, in addressing market failure, some who benefit from existing distortions will have an incentive to resist change, regardless of the wider social benefit. (Segal 2010)

Communities must also consider and debate the question of how much control should be vested in the state to legislate in matters that can be viewed as compromising democratic freedoms and the rights of free citizens. However, even where there is initial resistance, legislation that can demonstrate its benefits in protecting health can gain public acceptance *after* its introduction. For example, in 1990, the New South Wales government introduced the *Swimming Pools Act* to ensure that all residential pools were isolated from living areas and neighbouring property by a childproof fence. The Act was the first of its kind in Australia and was in the precarious position of setting an example for other states to follow. The Act also faced considerable opposition from special interest groups. However, after it was introduced, a survey by Elkington, Carey and Fowler (1992) found that, among pool owners, 85 per cent indicated that they approved of compulsory isolation-fencing and, even among pool owners yet to comply with the legislation, 70 per cent approved of the requirements.

CASE STUDY **8.4**

Pool fencing: a strategy for the reduction of child drowning deaths

Increasing affluence in Australia during the 1960s and 1970s resulted in the increase of home swimming pools and rising child drowning deaths. This saw local governments enact pool-fencing legislation, which was then taken up at a state or territory level. Initially, pool-fencing regulation only needed to restrict access from people outside the property, then it needed to be three-sided (no entry from the yard) and then four-sided (no direct entry to pool area from a building). In Australia in the last two decades there has been a decline in child drowning deaths largely attributed to pool fencing. However, a range of challenges is still present, including upgrading fencing to the latest standard and ensuring compliance with appropriate legislation.

In 2010 Queensland introduced legislation changes to improve pool safety, including that pools inspected at time of sale, when leased or sold and all new pools need four-sided fencing. In a 2011 randomised telephone survey, 1265 Queensland residents were asked, 'How effective do you think that tightening the pool-fencing legislation will be in reducing child drowning deaths?' Fifty-seven per cent of respondents believed that tightening pool-fencing legislation would be effective.

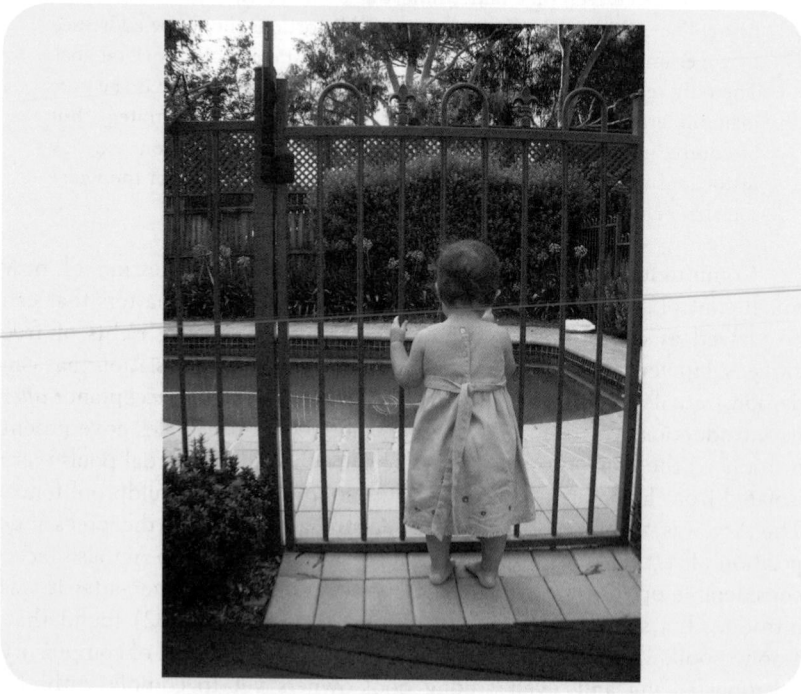

Photo courtesy of the Royal Life Saving Society Australia (www.royallifesaving.com.au).

While the number of children drowning in home swimming pools has decreased, there is still room for improvement. Despite concerted efforts, the message about pool fencing effectiveness does not appear to be reaching the most important group—pool owners. Better strategies to educate pool owners about the effectiveness of pool fence legislation, and to increase compliance, are required.

Franklin et al. 2012

At the micro-environmental level, in settings where health-promoting policies can be introduced, regulation can include local rules, protocols and policies that can have a profound effect on the health-related behaviour of individuals and organisations. Examples are school-based policies relating to food, which can influence options in school meals, vending machines and tuck shops, or changing instore product placement policy in supermarkets by placing fruit and vegetables instead of high fat and sugar snacks as potential last-minute 'impulse purchases' by shoppers at checkouts. The home is another important micro-setting where family rules about food purchase and consumption can alter the 'obesogenicity' of the home environment.

Ordinance changes can occur at the local government level as a result of lobbying, deputations, letter writing from local constituents, and community action. A now well-established technique for instituting action at the government level is the circulation of prepared forms for constituents to sign, send or email to local MPs and authorities. Because this removes two of the major barriers to individual action (i.e. time and effort), it can facilitate action.

Community plebiscites are another means of gaining support for local regulatory changes that can affect health, although these can sometimes be vulnerable to the undue influence of vocal minorities opposed to public health attempts at 'mass medication'. Community plebiscites have been strategically used by public health dentists in New South Wales to introduce fluoride to water supplies in rural towns (Sivaneswaran, Chong & Blinkhorn 2010).

Lobby groups and coalitions which are, or have been, effective in building momentum for legislative changes in health through consistent advocacy, and have more recently been using electronic media and strategies including e-petitions, e-referenda, e-citizen juries and other e-community tools, and sometimes social action (see Chapter 7) include:

* Action on Smoking and Health (ASH)
* The Nonsmokers' Rights Movement
* Billboard Utilising Graffitists Against Unhealthy Promotions (BUGAUP)
* Consumer's Health Forum
* People Against Drink Driving (PADD)
* Mothers Against Drink Driving (MADD)
* Australian Consumers Association (ACA)
* Australian Nutrition Foundation (ANF).

CASE STUDY **8.5**

**An example from the early days of legislation in health promotion:
'How will you go when you sit for the test?'**

The introduction of drinking restrictions on drivers in New South Wales in 1982, requiring a blood alcohol level of under 0.05 per cent, is an example of one of the most effective health promotion strategies of recent times, combining legislation and social marketing. Accompanying the introduction of the law was a strategically devised advertising campaign designed on the basis of qualitative research that indicated that drivers would *not* be influenced by appeals to social responsibility or fear of personal injury, but *were* concerned about the social embarrassment of being arrested.

**How will you go
when you sit for the test?**

**Will you be
under ·05 or under arrest?**

Random Breath Testing is in force throughout N.S.W.

The campaign—utilising a broadcast jingle and press, and bus sides and bumper stickers—used the slogan: *How will you go when you sit for the test? Will you be under .05 or under arrest?*

The combination of legislation and the media program (plus publicity generated) resulted in a 40 per cent decrease in traffic accidents in New South Wales in the first year of operation. However, a lack of visibility of breath testing units and lack of knowledge of people who had been arrested led to a decline in accident reductions in the second year of operation. This resulted in police later carrying out breath testing from more patrol cars, which were also more visible.

Bevins 1988

Technological interventions

Technological interventions are generally the domain of the medical, engineering or environmental expert. However, implementation and acceptance of such developments is often an opportunity for the health promotion practitioner to add value by placing the innovation in the context of a planned and evaluated health promotion program. The development of sunscreens to filter out the harmful effects of ultraviolet radiation, for example, has been a highly effective technological innovation, with health-beneficial consequences in the lives of many people who enjoy the beach and an outdoor lifestyle, particularly in Australia and New Zealand. A 10-year study by Dr Lawrence Greene and colleagues, of people who used sunscreens regularly versus a control group, found that long-term application of sunscreen decreases the risk of certain (potentially life-threatening) skin cancers (Greene et al. 2011). However, health promotion interventions are necessary to inform those at risk about the use of such sunscreens and to develop programs to counter social norms that inhibit the use of such innovations.

Because they do not rely on behaviour change alone for their effectiveness, technological interventions can also protect the health of the vulnerable, including the very young. For example, after community concerns and advocacy from public health groups, the US Product Standard Safety Commission enacted a new safety standard for child-resistant disposable cigarette lighters in 1997. A review of the effectiveness of this standard, which required that disposable cigarette lighters be resistant to operation by children younger than 5 years, found a 58 per cent reduction in fires attributable to this age group, preventing an estimated 100 deaths, 660 injuries and $52.5 million in property losses in 1998 alone (Smith, Green & Singh 2002).

In developing countries, technological interventions can also offer cost-effective health benefits where other strategies are not practical and/or new advances are pending. For example, while a malaria vaccine is still some years away, many people in low-lying areas of the tropical world are afforded a level of protection against disease-carrying mosquitoes through the use of insecticide-treated (bed) nets (Mouhamadou et al. 2006).

A wide range of workplace health and safety (WHS) devices (such as safety goggles, hoods over circular saws, and the wearing of protective helmets and boots) has added considerably to industrial and occupational safety. The reduction of noise through engineering techniques has been a major factor in the reduction of loss of hearing due to industrial and other noise. Contemporary WHS issues in office environments are likely to focus more closely on design to facilitate movement, lighting and ergonomic furniture, including standing workstations to address the potential health problems associated with prolonged sitting (see Owen et al. 2010).

The accelerating pace of technology shows no signs of slowing down in the twenty-first century. These innovations have sometimes provided mixed blessings for health—fast food and labour-saving home appliances being cases in point. However, it is the health promotion practitioner who may have the most crucial role to play in identifying the technologies that show most promise for health gain, and in building community support for their introduction and implementation. The use of home and gym-based exercise equipment, active entertainment such as television and electronic games powered by exercise bicycles, and activity sensors with devices for switching off electronics if enough movement is not carried out are examples of the use of technology to deal with the problems that technology has created (Egger, Swinburn & Rossner 2002). This will undoubtedly become a growth area in the future.

Organisational interventions

A major problem for health promotion is reaching the population that is targeted for intervention in sufficient numbers for the costs involved. For this reason, specific settings exist that enable greater access to 'captive' groups. This can include the workplace, schools, churches and other organisations and institutions where people gather.

Workplaces

The workplace provides a favourable framework for health promotion (Auvinen, Kohtamäki & Ilvesmäki 2012). There exists an infrastructure and organisation within workplaces for coordinating and developing programs that are more likely to be successful and of low cost (and therefore more sustainable) than programs without infrastructure.

In general, health promotion programs in the workplace are distinct and separate from the responsibilities that employers have in the implementation of proper occupational health and safety measures in the workplace. They include such activities as testing, health screening, ergonomics, education, provision of physical facilities such as fitness centres, ongoing health checks and occupational programs specific to particular industries.

Although the rationale for workplace health promotion would seem apparent, outcomes are not always so obvious. The provision of fitness facilities in many workplaces in Australia is often not successful, with these often only being used by a small number of dedicated staff (Corti 2001). Unlike the US, where corporations have a financial incentive for providing health services to staff, Australian corporations often have difficulty convincing staff that the workplace is more than a place to visit for a set time to complete their work requirements.

Workplace health promotion may also be condoned but not supported by a supervisor. Workers may feel coerced to participate by management. From a business perspective, both the direct and indirect costs of the program must be considered and those with influence in a corporation convinced that there are likely to be improvements resulting to the revenue base of the company. Workplace health promotion programs may create disruptions in work scheduling and can create employee-relations problems. For these and other reasons, results from evaluations of workplace health promotion interventions are often mixed (Cancelliere et al. 2011).

Despite these difficulties, health promotion in the workplace—by addressing deficits in knowledge, choice and social support in relation to a range of healthy behaviours—does hold promise for improving employee health, and has the potential to reduce social inequalities in health. A stimulus to this would be government and workplace regulations requiring minimum health promotion inputs for staff as part of occupational health requirements, a situation that already exists in some areas, such as providing workplace smoking policies and smoking cessation programs.

Health-promoting schools

School health promotion has grown significantly from a narrow concept focused on health instruction in the classroom to a much broader framework. Booth and Samdal (1997) characterise health-promoting schools under six domains, emphasising that, in practice, these domains of activity should be as thoroughly integrated as possible:

- the formal curriculum
- school ethos (the social environment)
- the physical environment
- the policies and practices of the school
- school health services
- the school–home–community interaction.

As might be anticipated, the adoption of a holistic health-promoting school concept is not achievable overnight. However, where implementation of programs is strategic and structured, gains can be made. A systematic review of the implementation and effectiveness of nutrition programs in schools (Wang & Stewart 2012) illustrates the following requirements for effectiveness:

- more professional training for teachers in the health-promoting schools approach
- further qualitative studies
- longer intervention periods
- improved follow-up evaluations
- adequate funding.

In another study aimed at looking at school policy effects on smoking in school children in Western Australia, Hamilton et al. (2003) found that the actions taken to deal with students who violate smoking policy restrictions may be more important in reducing cigarette smoking than the presence of health or drug policies or health committees. Using education/counselling and discipline strategies rather than discipline only may help to reduce teenage smoking, showing the benefits of a combined approach.

CASE STUDY **8.6**

Active-Ate: a program to promote health eating and activity in primary schools

The Active-Ate program, launched in 2004, was developed in North Queensland by Queensland Health and was delivered largely via an active website to Queensland primary schools, although some materials were delivered by mail. The program involved a wide range of activities summarised under the headings shown in the jigsaw below. What made Active-Ate particularly innovative was that it was not solely restricted to the classroom and included activities that involved the school and home environments. While it had been critically acclaimed as a best practice program in 2007, before its well-designed evaluation could be completed, Active-Ate was subsumed into the broader 'Smart Choices' set of initiatives to improve the supply of healthy food and drink choices in Queensland government schools. The demise of Active-Ate also provides a useful lesson for health promotion program developers: for programs to sustain over time there needs to be high level support and commitment from all stakeholders for project implementation and evaluation.

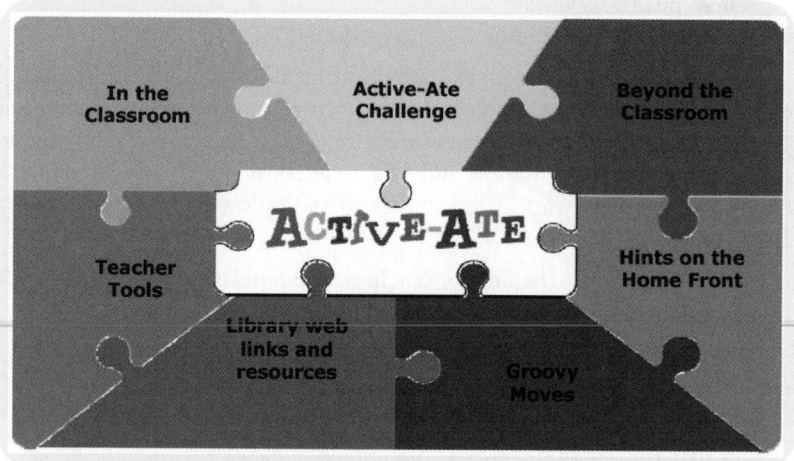

As has been observed with workplace health promotion, the development of valid evaluation instruments—to measure program implementation and to assess the effects of health-promoting school interventions—has lagged behind the development of conceptual and practical advances in this area (Booth & Samdal 1997). Nevertheless, the health-promoting schools movement is a global one, consistent with WHO principles (WHO 1995), and provides an opportunity to influence positively the health of a target group of unquestionable importance in our society—our children.

The use of incentives and disincentives

Stimulus–response learning theory implies that individual behaviour is learned as a result of positive and negative reinforcements. The use of incentives and disincentives, economic or otherwise, is a potential strategy in health promotion. Price manipulation is a simple, but obvious, example. Taxation changes to food products—both reductions and increases—may be expected to alter patterns of consumption of those foods. In particular, it is known that in bad economic times, the purchase of 'generic' food products increases and the sale of known brands decreases.

Price manipulations may have positive and negative implications for health. For example, public health nutritionists in north Queensland found that the cost of a 'healthy food basket' to feed an average family for one week that might be purchased in a remote Indigenous community store cost significantly more than the same basket in a metropolitan area. However, the cost of the 'unhealthy food basket' of soft drinks, biscuits and chips cost about the same, often due to food manufacturers subsidising the cost of freight of these products. These findings led to policy changes in government store policy in remote communities, which included freight subsidies for fresh fruit and vegetables and a range of other 'best buys' for improved nutrition for Aboriginal and Torres Strait Islander populations (Lee et al. 2009).

Manipulation at the point of sale is an option that is relatively unused by nutritionists—even though commercial research shows that up to 50 per cent of food-sale decisions is made at this point. Further incentives in food purchase include the introduction of endorsements on packaging by health bodies such as the Heart Foundation's 'Pick the Tick' program (Williams, McMahon & Boustead 2003).

Changes in demand for substances such as alcohol and tobacco can also be significantly affected by price increases resulting from sales and excise taxes. Australia is unique in its funding of health promotion programs in several states through a special levy on tobacco.

Major changes in taxation policy obviously require detailed negotiations. Introduction of tax changes is difficult for governments that are concerned about possible electoral backlash. At the local level, the health promotion practitioner can facilitate incentives—such as in local food outlets. Approaches can be made to cooperative supermarket managers with the incentive of increasing sales of healthy foods (e.g. fruits and vegetables, breakfast cereals, low-fat dairy products), through such initiatives as:

- instore promotions
- having a nutritionist on the spot
- changing point-of-sale materials.

Manufacturers are also often keen to be involved in promotions that positively affect the sales of their products. Increased interest in health in recent times has created a market for the development of products specifically with a health orientation.

Economic incentives have also been used with individuals to:

- encourage smokers at the workplace to quit smoking
- reduce sickness absenteeism
- help people lose weight
- be involved in workplace health programs.

CASE STUDY 8.7

Using incentives to create change: The Norfolk Island Carbon and Health Evaluation (NICHE) program

Using the principle that climate change and obesity may have a common cause (i.e. increased fossil fuel use and inactivity and high energy-dense food production and high calorie intake), the Norfolk Island Carbon and health Evaluation (NICHE) trial is a world-first study testing the theory that people who reduce their carbon footprint might also decrease their rates of obesity.

Carbon trading is being considered as a means of reducing greenhouse gas emissions and their environmental effects. To date, attention has focused primarily on a carbon tax, to provide 'upstream' reductions in emissions. However, 40–60 per cent of emissions come from individuals and households. This has led to proposals for a more 'downstream' system involving personal carbon trading (PCT). In addition to modifying greenhouse gas emissions (and particularly carbon), PCT has been suggested as a possible way of improving health, in particular by reducing obesity and chronic diseases, such as type 2 diabetes.

The NICHE program is a world-first study to test this in a relatively closed (e.g. island) system over a three-year period. The proposal has been developed by three Australian universities, based on proposals developed initially in the UK, the main goal being to test attitudes (and hence acceptability) of an incentive scheme for saving energy and reducing a community's carbon footprint. Another goal is to test the theory that if individuals become more environmentally conscious this can have a positive impact on their health through better health behaviours (i.e. more exercise and healthy diet). (See www.niche.nlk.nf.)

Egger 2007

Sponsorship

Health promotion professionals around the globe have adopted many of the concepts and tools of commercial marketing. However, it has been mainly in Australia and New Zealand that health-promoting organisations have adopted sponsorship strategies, both as sponsors (mainly government agencies) and by actively promoting themselves to business as sponsees (non-government agencies). This has been facilitated by the fact that small scale sponsorships at selected events are within the capacity of even small agencies to implement and by a growing awareness among health and sporting organisations of the 'natural' fit between both types of organisations' goals. The greater congruence between the sponsor and the sponsee on some overall characteristics (what is called the sponsor 'fit'), the more effective will be the sponsorship (Alay 2008; Rifon et al. 2004). Red Bull's sponsorship of UK Athletics (UKA) as the 'official drink to UKA' is an example of 'good fit'. Under the sponsorship, Red Bull has exclusive rights to provide energy drinks and drink stations across UKA offices, to coaching staff, training camps, conferences and squads. Red Bull will also provide products at all UKA competitions and have a strong field presence at all UKA televised events (SportBusiness International 2009).

Sponsorship is generally defined as payment for the right to associate the sponsor's company name, products or services with a 'sponsee' in return for various promotional benefits to the sponsor. The sponsee may be:

- an organisation—for example, the NHF being sponsored by a drug company
- an event—for example, a triathalon
- a series of events—for example, a theatre season
- an individual—for example, a prominent sports person
- a group of individuals—for example, an AFL team.

Many high-profile commercial sponsorships are accompanied by extensive promotional activities—such as mass media advertising, product samplings, trade promotions and exclusive merchandising agreements.

Sponsorship is considered to offer a number of benefits or opportunities to the sponsor:

- the ability to cost-effectively reach specific target audiences with little 'wastage' on persons outside the target group (e.g. young people at rock concerts, joggers at a fun run)
- the opportunity for potential trial of the sponsor's product where the sponsorship includes exclusive stocking agreements (e.g. a soft drink or snack-food marketer)
- hospitality for clients, employees and other stakeholders

- the generation of community goodwill by sponsoring not-for-profit organisations popular with the community
- enhanced communication effects such as increased company profile, increased brand awareness, and brand-image formation or reinforcement associated with positive attributes of the sponsored event or individual (Sweeney 2002).

CASE STUDY **8.8**

Sponsorship and the health promotion foundations: the case of Healthway

The advent of tobacco tax-funded health promotion foundations is a relatively new phenomenon in public health theory and practice. In Australia, foundations now exist in two states—the first (VicHealth) having been established in 1987 in Victoria. Interest in the concept of health promotion foundations is now spreading to other parts of the globe and Carroll (2003) has now documented the Australian and overseas experiences for adoption in other countries.

Although the two Australian foundations are different, the following description of the Western Australian Health Promotion Foundation (known as 'Healthway') illustrates the principal concepts. Healthway was established in 1991 under tobacco-control legislation that outlawed the public promotion of tobacco products. Healthway is funded by a levy raised on the wholesale distribution of tobacco products. It uses approximately 60 per cent of its funds to sponsor Sport, Arts and Racing Groups (SARGs). SARGs may range from one-off small craft exhibitions to a series of state theatre plays, or from coaching clinics for junior soccer players to professional league teams such as Australian Football League and National Basketball League teams.

When Healthway provides sponsorship funds (a 'grant') to a SARG, it simultaneously awards support funds to an independent health agency to promote a health message at the sport, arts or racing event. Health organisations (e.g. the Heart Foundation, Cancer Foundation, Diabetes Association) and their messages (e.g. 'Be Smokefree', 'Be Active Every Day', 'Eat More Fruit and Veg.', 'Be Sun Wise', 'Drinksafe'; 'Act–Belong–Commit') are chosen primarily with respect to the nature of the particular event's audience or participants, and with respect to the state's health priority areas. For very small grants, and especially for country SARGs, rather than allocating funds to a health agency, Healthway provides the SARG with a sponsorship support 'kit' containing posters, decals, pamphlets and ideas for activities with respect to a specific health message.

Healthway also attempts to create healthy environments within clubs and at events by negotiating the introduction of smokefree areas, availability of low-alcohol and non-alcohol alternatives, safe alcohol-serving practices, provision of healthy food choices and sun-protection measures (such as shaded spectator areas and protective clothing). These initiatives are the equivalent of merchandising and stocking agreements in commercial sponsorship.

In 2010, Healthway formally adopted a policy of requiring organisations that accepted Healthway sponsorship to not accept sponsorship by alcohol and unhealthy food marketers. This co-sponsorship policy supports the objective of the sponsorship program to reduce, where possible, the promotion of unhealthy messages or brands that undermine Healthway objectives. (See www.healthway. wa.gov.au.)

Carroll 2003

The sponsee also benefits in a number of ways, including the raising of its profile in the community—an important benefit for non-profit organisations' fundraising efforts—and the attraction of members or volunteers. For sponsored health organisations, the major benefits are the increased ability to promote their health messages to a larger number of people, and to reach target audiences who might not otherwise be reached (Corti et al. 1997).

In most countries, total sponsorship expenditure is still small relative to other marketing expenditure, but this figure is increasing and is expected to grow at an increasing rate. Growth is being fuelled by the increased costs of media and other promotions, and by the apparent cost-effectiveness of sponsorship—at least in terms of delivering media exposure of the sponsor's brand name or logo for a minimal outlay.

The entry of large companies into sponsorship programs has also been stimulated by non-profit organisations actively promoting themselves as vehicles for sponsorship (e.g. the Australian Institute of Sport and Kellogg's 'Sustain' and the Heart Foundation's 'tick' labelling).

Sponsorship, particularly of sport, received major impetus in Australia as a result of the tobacco companies seeking ways to continue to promote their brands following bans on television advertising and, later, on other forms of promotion. Given the tobacco companies' apparent success in maintaining brand awareness and image via sponsorship, other companies—led by the major brewery and soft drink marketers—increasingly have included sponsorship as part of their promotional mix.

During this same period, health promotion professionals adopted many of the concepts and tools of commercial marketing, and now are enthusiastically embracing sponsorship.

The growth in health sponsorship has been facilitated in Australia primarily by the health promotion foundations. The growth in health sponsorship has been facilitated further by the deliberate policy in some states of guaranteeing the replacement of tobacco sponsorship funds with health promotion foundation funds following the legislative phasing out of tobacco sponsorship. The replacement of tobacco sponsorship with health sponsorship has occurred elsewhere, for example, in California (see Weinreich, Abbott & Olsen 1999); health sponsorship as a strategy has been adopted in New Zealand (via the Health Sponsorship Council; see www.hsc.org.nz) and in Canada (via Health Canada; see O'Reilly and Madill 2007).

Does sponsorship work?

While much sponsorship evaluation is commercial-in-confidence, there are many published studies and business reports to show that sponsorship can be very effective in reaching and impacting its target audiences. With respect to health sponsorships, in January 1992, the University of Western Australia was commissioned by Healthway to undertake the Health Promotion Development and Evaluation Program (HPDEP) over three years. HPDEP, a joint undertaking of the Graduate School of Management and the Department of Public Health, is now known as the Health Promotion Evaluation Unit (HPEU). Through HPDEP/HPEU, Healthway has carried out extensive evaluation of its sponsorship activities. Generally, these evaluations show that sponsorship can be effective in increasing awareness of health messages and in creating intentions to adopt healthy behaviours (Donovan & Henley 2010).

A healthy environment—ecological considerations

The union of health promotion and concern for the natural environment is an idea whose time has come. Environmental changes have traditionally been one of the cornerstones of public health—the provision of potable water, garbage disposal and sanitation. In the past, these modifications have been to a hostile natural environment which Western tradition has felt obliged to 'tame'. Ironically, when this appears to have been achieved, the environment has fought back in an unexpected and potentially more dangerous way.

Dubos (1988) expressed his concern for humanity's current predicament in the following way:

> In short, the two worlds of man—the biosphere of his inheritance, the technosphere of his creation—are out of balance, indeed potentially in deep conflict. And man is in the middle. This is the hinge of history at which we stand, the door of the future opening on to a crisis more sudden, more global, more inescapable, and more bewildering than any ever encountered by the human species and one which will take decisive shape within the life span of children who are already born.

Environmental degradation, pollution, the 'greenhouse effect', disappearance of the ozone layer and the disruption of the planet's ecosystems

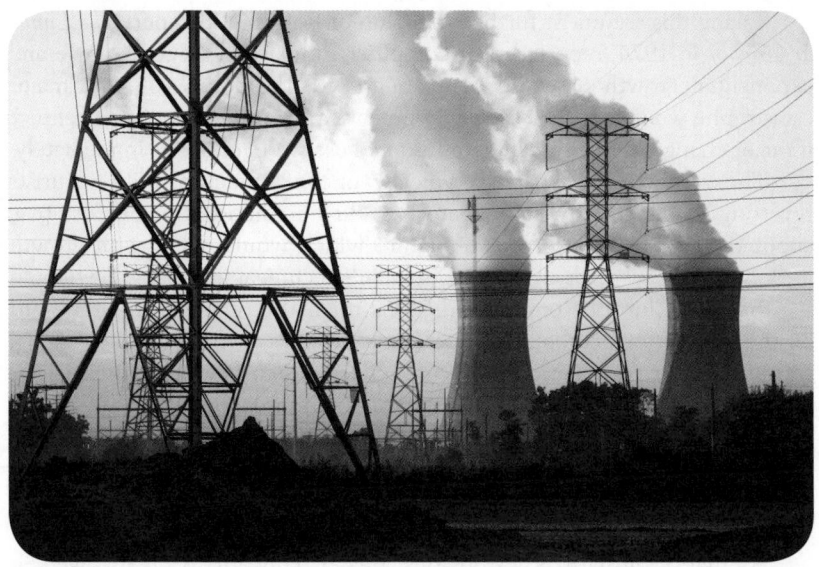

have all become apparent as a result of attempts to improve living standards. They pose future challenges not only to scientists and politicians, but also to health workers and educationalists. After all, it is likely to be changes in human behaviour—in population growth, resource use and economic activity—that will stop environmental degradation over the long term. To this end, the health promotion practitioner of the future is likely to work with environmentalists, engineers and ecologists.

Without close consideration, it might be expected that the contributions of health science and technological development to humanity would all be positive. In his epic novel *Brave New World*, Aldous Huxley described this as 'the myth of progress'. In essence, Huxley saw all medical and scientific advances as a danger to the human race because each of these promotes the survival and propagation of the biologically and genetically unfit. These advances then negate the forces of natural selection and may ultimately be responsible for the fall of humanity.

As early as 1964, the US economist Kenneth Boulding related the development of negative returns in health to the exponential growth of human populations:

> [I]f the only thing which can check the growth of population is starvation and misery, then the population will grow until it is sufficiently miserable and starving to check its own growth. (Boulding 1964)

Boulding also noted, somewhat facetiously, that: 'Anyone who believes that exponential growth can continue forever, is either a madman or an Economist.'

Taking this argument further, the Club of Rome, in its report *The Limits to Growth* in 1974, reported on a computer simulation of energy usage and exponential growth of world population, with the conclusion that major catastrophe would occur to the environment early in the twenty-first century if major changes in the direction of resource use were not made immediately.

The response to this was typically one of cynicism, with futurists reverting to history to demonstrate that dire predictions in the past (e.g. about the proliferation of horse manure which would occur with growth in population) were always solved by man's technical ingenuity. Few could see that the Club of Rome's predictions might be reflected in alterations in the ozone and carbon dioxide levels in the environment, or global warming in the time period predicted—all of which have the potential for major changes in the world's environment and human health. In any case, a 30-year update of the Club of Rome data (Meadows, Randers & Meadows 2004) has shown that the developments in world pollution are on track with a 'business as usual' model, as predicted in the 1974 report, and this has been supported by other, independent modelling (Turner 2008).

Population growth is an obvious area of concern to all involved in human health and services. Whereas it took from the beginning of man's time on earth to 1850 for the world population to reach 1 billion, it required only another 100 years for that number to double. On present trends, the number will double again in the first two decades of the twenty-first century. And, although population growth has slowed in the developed world, there is no indication of this in those parts of the world where demand for the earth's resources has yet to increase. Population control and family planning will obviously become a major role for the preventive-health worker of the future. This poses a range of religious, philosophical and democratic challenges, which will need to be addressed.

However, population growth alone may be merely a symptom of a more deep-seated and insidious cause. The drive for economic growth at an exponential rate—which is required in current Western economies—means either that more resources must be consumed per person, more people must exist to consume more resources or new resources must be discovered or produced more efficiently. The combination of resource depletion and population growth creates an environmental time bomb that may eventually require a major paradigm shift in the way in which we live. As pointed out by one writer:

> We have dallied too long at the banquet of natural resources, only to discover that the only way out is past the cashier. Even among those who are aware of the scale of our environmental debt, the general consensus seems to be that with the aid of a little fast technological tap dancing most of us may make our escape without paying the full price. Not only would this involve a drastic and immediate reduction in the daily rate at which we

gobble up the world's energy resources and dump our wastes, but we would have to sacrifice two of western civilizations most sacred cows—Growth and Progress—to do it. (Morrison 2003)

In a study of the distal causes of obesity, Egger and Swinburn (2011; Egger, Swinburn and Islam 2012) concluded that a 'sweet spot' for growth has now passed and that we are now achieving negative returns in terms of declining health as a result of unfettered economic growth—and increasing wealth in a unequal society.

A new challenge for health promotion in the twenty-first century will be dealing with the consequences of the ecological disruptions that are already occurring throughout the world. This was summed up eloquently by Australian epidemiologist, Dr Tony McMichael, as early as 1992:

> [A] new and unfamiliar public health hazard is emerging. The fact that the hazard is neither immediate nor tangible is part of the problem. This is a qualitatively different category of public health problem from those previously encountered. Much of it is global in scope; it does not depend on directly acting environmental exposures; it transcends generations; and some aspects may be irreversible. It includes global warming and its many ecological consequences, increased exposure to biologically damaging ultra-violet radiation, loss of arable land, destruction of parts of our food chain, loss of biodiversity, and urban crowding and social disintegration. While there is much that is uncertain and controversial, there is little doubt that recent trends and their implications for human health are troubling. (McMichael 1992).

McMichael's warning is not a doomsday prophecy. He observes that an ecological transition to a sustainable society can be achieved if we breathe life into the much-parroted phrase 'our common future':

> The stabilisation of resource use, and of human numbers, will require radical reforms of our core values, economic priorities and structures—and of social decision-making processes. It will require governments, private enterprise, non-government organisations, communities and economists—we're all in this together. (McMichael & Hales 1997)

Furthermore, as we undertake some of the above reforms we should not underestimate the role of public health measures in combating at least some of the problems that we face. For example, some authorities have expressed concern that all the attention to global warming as a public health problem could distract the public from other, more urgent, health priorities. On the other hand, as discussed earlier, it may provide a 'stealth intervention' for dealing with the bigger problems facing the world (Egger 2012). Involving the business community, who stand to profit from maintenance of the status quo, will be the key issue. Cooperation of futuristic thinkers in this area, like entrepreneur and former Australian of the Year Dick Smith (2011), will be vital for the health promotion of the future.

Implications for the health promotion practitioner

How can the health promotion practitioner influence such broad issues as the environment and its degradation? In the first place, health promotion skills can assist with awareness of the problem as it relates to health. Media acceptance of environmental problems has now allowed a forum for this discussion to take place. For example, Selvey and Carey have recently called for greater use of an 'environmental lens' in examining some of our public health policy cornerstones such as the Australian Dietary Guidelines. In a recent critique of the latest draft guidelines they note that recommendations, for example, to increase drinking water and fish in the diet, may be nutritionally sound but need to consider the impact of disposable water bottles on the environment and the critical state of Australian (and global) fish stocks (Selvey & Carey 2013).

The relationship of environmental issues to health is apparent in obvious ways (e.g. exposure to sunlight and potential increases in skin cancer), but also in less obvious ways (e.g. pollution). Awareness needs to be translated into knowledge, which can be converted into action. This requires action at all levels of intervention—using media, community organisation and community development—in an approach incorporating *global* not just *local* thinking. Action may not simply involve changing individual behaviour but may involve mobilising community interest groups on the side of a health-promoting environment and against entrenched and powerful opposition such as non-renewable resource industries.

CASE STUDY **8.9**

A 10-point checklist for healthy and sustainable communities

It has been argued that all human development should consider these factors:

1. Outdoor air quality—through reduced dependence on motor vehicles and reduced pollution
2. Water supply and sanitation
3. Housing and buildings—with implications for human health (e.g. solar powered, ventilation, avoidance of chemicals)
4. Food—including urban agriculture and access to local supplies
5. Local shops and services
6. Schools and other educational institutions
7. Community spaces—for recreation and social interaction
8. Transport and street connectivity—encouraging cycling and walking
9. Communication technology—including high speed internet services
10. Economy and employment (with e.g. reduced commuting times)

Capon & Blakely 2007

Methods for modifying the health environment

Because the role of the health promotion practitioner in environmental interventions has no well-defined professional precedents, there are no clear rules of operation. However, some principles include the following:

- investigation and communication concerning local environmental issues and problems that impact on health, political lobbying—at the local as well as national and state levels
- letter writing—including deputation-style letters for constituents' signatures
- community organisation—at several levels of involvement
- community development—particularly among affected groups and individuals
- awareness raising—by use of media, public forums, lectures, organised debates, article writing, publicity and festivals
- demonstration–participation programs—for example, clean-ups, smoke-outs, live-ins
- cooperation with local retailers, wholesalers, and manufacturers for mutually advantageous gains, including sponsorships.

Summary of environmental approaches

Manipulations of the health environment often represent the greatest challenge to the health practitioner, but can also be the most cost-effective and time-effective processes for influencing health behaviour. Even though the focus is macro-level change, the issues at stake pose considerably greater potential risk to life and health for the community than do individual risk factors.

Because the basis of much ill-health in modern times lies in structural and socio-political causes, it is important for the health promotion practitioner to attempt to modify these causes at the local or national level. The Greenpeace motto 'Think Globally, Act Locally' is an apt principle for operation at this level. Doing so may involve the use of any or all of the strategies outlined above. But it may also involve a creative approach to more direct action.

Career opportunities in health promotion

Environmental interventions have always been a part of effective public health, albeit from a different perspective than is required today. Health promotion practitioners have potential opportunities in policy settings, in designing physical environments that promote health, from careers such as town and community planners, architecture and engineering, to designing, promoting and selling 'active technology' like fitness equipment and active games. Political advocacy and political lobbying, particularly in environmental agencies or NGOs offer other opportunities,

continued

continued

as does employment as environmental health or sport and recreation officers with local or state governments. Opportunities in education are also expanding in the area of health and physical education in schools and as nutrition consultants and advisers with schools and education departments. Health promotion personnel working in community development or family planning also stimulate much environmental change, particularly within aid and humanitarian assistance organisations in developing countries. Specialists in injury prevention and public health are often required to also have a background in health promotion.

References

Alay, S., 2008, Female consumers' evaluations of sponsorship and their response to sponsorship, *South African J Res Sport, Physical Educ Recreat* 30(2):15–29.

Auvinen, A.M., Kohtamäki K., & Ilvesmäki, A., 2012, Workplace health promotion and stakeholder positions: a Finnish case study, *Arch Environ Occup Health* 67(3):177–84.

Bergenstal, J., Davis S.M., Sikora R., Paulson D., & Whiteman C., 2012, Pediatric bicycle injury prevention and the effect of helmet use: the West Virginia experience, *West Virginia Med J* 108(3):78–81.

Bevins, J., 1988, Reducing communication abuse, Paper presented to the Fourth Drug Education Conference, Perth, Western Australia.

Bierer, M.F., & Rigotti, N.A., 1992, Public policy for the control of tobacco-related disease, *Clin Med North Am* 76:515–39.

Booth, M.L., & Samdal, O., 1997, Health-promoting schools in Australia: models and measurement, *Aust N Z J Public Health* 21(4):365–70.

Boulding, K., 1964, *The Meaning of the Twentieth Century*, Harper & Row, New York.

Brownell, K.D., 2004, *Food Fight*, Contemporary Books, New York.

Cancelliere, C., Cassidy J.D., Ammendolia C., & Côté P., 2011, Are workplace health promotion programs effective at improving presenteeism in workers? A systematic review and best evidence synthesis of the literature, *BMC Public Health* May 26;11:395.

Capon, A.G., & Blakely E.J., 2007, Checklist for health and sustainable communities, *NSW Public Health Bull* 18(3–4):51–4.

Carroll, A., 2003, The Western Australian Health Promotion Foundation—Healthway, *Health Promot J Aust* 1993; 3:42–3.

Chapman S., 2004, Public Health Advocacy, in Moodie R., & Hulme, A. (Eds), *Hands on Health Promotion*, IP Communications, Melbourne.

Club of Rome, 1974, *The Limits To Growth*, Universe Books, New York.

Corti, B., 2001, *Workplace Fitness*, In National Physical Activity Guidelines, Background Data, National Health and Medical Research Council, Canberra.

Corti, B., Holman, C.D.J., Donovan, R.J., Frizzell, S.K., & Caroll, A.M., 1997, Using sponsorship to promote health messages to children, *Health Educ & Behav* 24(3):276–86.

Daube, M., 2012, *Defending prevention—a battle we cannot afford to lose*, A speech to the Media Health Club, Brisbane, 4 August.

Donovan, R.J., & Henley, N., 2010, *Social Marketing: Principles and Practice*, (2nd ed) IP Communications, Melbourne.

Dubos, R., 1988, *Only One Earth*, Doubleday, London.

Dunnette, D.A., 1989, Cooking dinner while the house is burning: an environmental scientist's view of health education needs for the 1990s, *Health Ed* 20(7):4–7.

Egger, G., 2007, Personal carbon trading: a potential 'stealth intervention' for obesity reduction?, *Med J Aust* 187:185–7.

Egger, G., 2012, Health and sustainability, in Murray, J. et al. (Eds), *Enough for All Forever: A Handbook for Learning About Sustainability*, Common Ground Publishing, Champaigne, Illinois.

Egger, G., & Swinburn, B., 1997, An ecological approach to the obesity pandemic, *BMJ* 315:477–80.

Egger G., & Swinburn B., 2011, *Planet Obesity: How we are eating ourselves and the planet to death*, Allen & Unwin, Sydney.

Egger, G., & Swinburn, B., 2013, Prevention of obesity in adults, in Bouchard, C. et al. (Eds), *Handbook of Obesity* (3rd edn), Human Kinetics, New York (in press).

Egger G., Swinburn B., & Islam A., 2012, Economic growth and obesity: a dynamic relationship with interesting implications, *Econ Human Biol* 10(2):147–53.

Egger, G., Swinburn, B., & Rossner, S., 2002, Dusting off the epidemiological triad: could it work with obesity? *Obes Rev* 3:289–301.

Elkington, J.M., Carey, V., & Fowler, D., 1992, Public perceptions of the New South Wales pool fencing legislation, *Health Prom J Aust* 2(1):34–7.

Franklin, R.C., Peden, A., Watt, K., & Leggat, P., 2012, Pool fencing: can Australia go much further?, Paper presented to Safety 2012, 11th World Conference on Injury Prevention and Safety Promotion, Wellington , New Zealand, 1–4 October.

Greene, A.C., Williams, G.A., Logan, V., & Strutton, G.M., 2011, Reduced melanoma after regular sunscreen use: randomized trial follow-up, *J Am Soc Clinical Oncol* 29(3):257–63.

Haddon W., 1980, Advances in the epidemiology of injuries as a basis for public policy, *Public Health Reports* 95(5):411–20.

Hamilton, G., Cross, D., Lower, T., Resnicow, K., & Williams, P., 2003, School policy: what helps to reduce teenage smoking? *Nicotine Tob Res* 4:507–13.

Higgins, D.N., Tierney, J., & Hanrahan, L., 2002, Preventing young worker fatalities. The Fatality Assessment and Control Evaluation (FACE) Program, *AAOHN J* 50(11):508–14.

Howland, J., & Rohsenhow, D.J., 2013, Risks of energy drinks mixed with alcohol, *JAMA* 309(3):245–6.

IUATLD (International Union Against Tuberculosis and Lung Disease), 2007, *Effective Mass Media Campaigns for Tobacco Control: Campaign Profile No. 18—'Nobody Smokes Here Anymore'*, Paris, available at www.theunion.org.

Kendrick, D., Young B., & Mason-Jones A.J. et al., 2012, Home safety education and provision of safety equipment for injury prevention, *Cochrane Database Syst Rev* Sep 12;9, CD005014.

Lee, A.J., Leonard, D., Moloney, A.A., & Mnniecon, D., 2009, Improving Aboriginal and Torres Strait Islander nutrition and health, *Med J Aust* 150(10):547–8.

McMichael, A., 1992, Ecological disruption and human health: the next great challenge to public health, *Aust J Public Health* 16(1):3–5.

McMichael, A., & Hales, S., 1997, Global health promotion: looking back to the future, *Aust NZ J Public Health* 21(4):425–8.

Meadows, D., Randers, J., & Meadows, D., 2004, *Limits to Growth: The 30 Year Update*, Chelsea Green Publishing, New York.

Mock, C., Quansah, R., Krishnan, R., Arreola-Risa, C., & Rivara, F., 2004, Strengthening the prevention and care of injuries worldwide, *Lancet* 363:2172–9.

Morley-John, J., Swinburn, B., Metcalf, P., Raza, F., & Wright, H., 2002, Fat content of chips, quality of frying fat and deep-frying practices in New Zealand fast food outlets, *Aust N Z J Public Health* 26:101–7.

Morrison R., 2003, *Plague Species: Is It in Our Genes?*, Reed New Holland, Sydney.

Mouhamadou, C., Simard, F., Chandre, F., Etang, J., Darriet, F., & Hougard, J.M., 2006, The efficacy of bifenthrin-impregnated bednets against Anopheles funestus and pyrethroid-resistant Anopheles gambiae in North Cameroon, *Malaria J* 5:77.

NPHT (National Preventative Health Taskforce), 2009, *Australia: the Healthiest Country by 2020—National Preventative Health Strategy*, Commonwealth of Australia, Canberra.

Ooi, E., Kee-Tai, G., & Gubler, D.J., 2006, Dengue prevention and 35 years of vector control in Singapore, *Emerg Infect Dis* June; 12(6):887–93.

O'Reilly, N., & Madill, J., 2007, Evaluating social marketing elements in sponsorship, *Soc Marketing Quarterly* 13(4):1–25.

Owen, N., Healy, G.N., Matthews, C.E., & Dunstan, D.W., 2010, Too much sitting: the population health science of sedentary behaviour, *Exerc Sci Rev* 38 (3):105–13.

Page Y., Cuny S., Hermitte T., & Labrousee M., 2012, A comprehensive overview of the frequency and the severity of injuries sustained by car occupants and subsequent implications in terms of injury prevention, *Ann Adv Automot Med* 56:165–74.

Pearson, T.A., 2011, Public policy approaches to the prevention of heart disease and stroke, *J Am Heart Assoc* 124:2560–71.

Penman, A., 2008, Regulation for chronic disease control: the pathfinder role of tobacco, *NSW Public Health Bull* 19(11–12):195–8.

Rifon, N., Choi, S., Trimble, C., & Li, H., 2004, Congruence effects in sponsorship: the mediating role of sponsor credibility and consumer attributions of sponsor motive, *J Advertising* 33(1),29–42.

Robinson, T.N., & Sirard, J.R., 2005, Preventing childhood obesity: a solution-oriented research paradigm, *Am J Prev Med* 28(2 Suppl 2):194–201.

Segal, L., 2010, The role of government in preventive health: 'nanny state' or redressing market and policy decisions, *Aust Med (online)*, 5 April, available at www.ausmed.ama.com.au.

Selvey, L.A., & Carey, M.G., 2013, Australia's dietary guidelines and the environmental impact of food from paddock to plate, *Med J Aust* 198(1):1–2.

Sepkowitz, K.A., 2013, Energy drinks and caffeine-related adverse effects, *JAMA* 309(3):243–4.

Simmons, A., Mavoa, H.M., Bell, A.C., de Courten, M., Schaaf, D., Schultz, J., & Swinburn, B.A., 2009, Creating community action plans for obesity prevention using the ANGELO (Analysis Grid for Elements Leading to Obesity), *Health Promot Int* 24(4): 311–24.

Sivaneswaran, S., Chong, G., & Blinkhorn, A., 2010, Successful fluoride plebiscite in the township of Deniliquin, New South Wales, Australia, *J Public Health Dentist* 70:163–6.

Sleet, D., 1990, Injury prevention, Seminar presentation to the Western Australian Professional Health Education Association (WAPHEA), Perth, May.

Smith, L., Greene, M., & Singh, H., 2002, A study of the effectiveness of the US safety standard for child-resistant cigarette lighters, *Inj Prev* 8:192–6.

Smith, R., 2011, *Dick Smith's Population Crisis*, Allen & Unwin, Sydney.

SportBusiness International, 2009, Red Bull extends UK athletics partnership, *SportBusiness*.

Sweeney, B., 2002, *Australians and Sport*, Brian Sweeney & Associates, Melbourne.

Swinburn, B., 2002, Influencing environments to reduce obesity prevalence, Plenary paper presented to the 9th International Congress on Obesity, Sao Paulo, Brazil 24–29 August.

Swinburn, B., Egger, G., & Raza, F., 1999, Dissecting obesogenic environments: Part of a public health approach to reducing obesity, *Prev Med* 29:563–70.

Thompson, D., & Rivara, F., 2003 Pool fencing for preventing drowning in children, *Cochrane Database Syst Rev* 1: CD001047.

Turner, G., 2008, A comparison of the limits to growth with 30 years of reality, *Global Environ Change* 18:397–411.

Vogels, N., Egger, G., Plasqi, G., & Westerterp, K.R., 2004, Estimating changes in daily physical activity levels over time: Implications for health interventions from a novel approach, *Int J Sports Med* 25: 607–10.

Wang, G., Macera, C.A., Scudder-Soucie, B., Schmid, T., Pratt, M., & Buchner, D., 2005, A cost-benefit analysis of physical activity using bike/pedestrian trails, *Health Promot Pract* April; 6(2):174–8.

Wang, D., & Stewart, D., 2012, The implementation and effectiveness of school-based nutrition promotion programmes using a health-promoting schools approach: a systematic review, *Public Health Nutr* Jul 31:1–19[Epub ahead of print].

Weinreich, N.K., Abbott, J., & Olson, C.K., 1999, Social marketers in the driver's seat: motorsport sponsorship as a vehicle for tobacco prevention, *Social Marketing Quarterly*, 5(3): 108–12.

Williams P., McMahon A., & Boustead R., 2003, A case study of sodium reduction in breakfast cereals and the impact of the Pick the Tick food information program in Australia, *Health Promot Int* Mar;18(1):51–6.

WHO, 1995, *WHO Expert Committee on Comprehensive School Health Education and Promotion*, WHO, Geneva.

WHO, 1986, *Ottawa Charter for Health Promotion*, International Conference on Health Promotion, Ottawa.

Wu, F., 2012, Advancing knowledge on the environment and its impact on health, and meeting the challenges of global environmental change, *Environ Health Perspect* 120(12):a450.

Zatonski, W.A., & Willett, W., 2005, Changes in dietary fat and declining coronary heart disease in Poland: population-based study, *BMJ* 331:187–8.

chapter **9**

Factors influencing strategy selection

Summary of main points

- The selection of the most appropriate strategy in health promotion can depend on a range of factors including the intended recipients, temporal factors, program factors and the level of community acceptance and participation.
- Strategy selection can also be influenced by the rate at which ideas are diffused among an intended audience.
- Different strategies may be needed to reach audiences with low economic resources and high risk.
- Although a single strategy may be applicable in particular circumstances, combinations of strategies are usually required.
- Health promotion strategies that ignore the deeper social causes of ill-health are unlikely to be successful over the long term.
- Obtaining ongoing funding for health promotion will generally be dependent on evidence from some level of evaluation being demonstrated.

The story so far

An understanding of all the processes discussed to this point in this book should lead to the following conclusions:

- The professional health promotion practitioner, by necessity, needs to be a 'specialist in generalisation'.
- Knowledge is required in both the *content* of health issues and the *processes* by which change can be instigated to attain health improvement.

- Due to the multifactorial nature of this field and the evidence that for most (but not all) situations and health issues, a range of complementary strategies is more likely to be effective than a single strategy, the three most common words in discussing the relevance of health promotion strategies are '*it all depends*'.
- The role of the health promotion practitioner is often that of a translator (translating information from the scientific community to the general public), a moderator, a facilitator, and/or a catalyst for action.
- Understanding one's limitations and developing one's skills in the range of strategies available are of prime professional concern to the health promotion practitioner.
- Strategies for coping with individual risk are important, but strategies dealing with lowering average risk in whole communities and addressing underlying social inequities—as well as physical and lifestyle risk factors that predispose to ill-health—are likely to be more effective in the long term.
- Combinations of strategies and methods are likely to yield the best results.

The approach of this text has been based on strategies and methods rather than settings or health issues. The application of strategies and methods to settings requires the knowledge and experience of the practitioner and an appreciation of the needs of the target group. For example:

- *School-based programs*—can include the lecture–discussion format and any or all of the different group methods or broader health-promoting schools approaches.
- *Primary health care*—might include one-to-one health education, screening and early detection and is increasingly a setting where health promotion is integrated into primary healthcare practice with an emphasis on community partnerships (e.g. see the Integrated Health Promotion Resource Kit from the Victorian Department of Human Services, www.health.vic.gov.au/healthpromotion).
- *Workplace programs*—may call for group techniques, plus risk factor analysis and changes to the workplace environment (such as workstations and healthy canteens).
- *Institution-based programs* (e.g. hospitals, aged-care facilities)—could involve in-hospital group and individual programs as well as community organisation or outreach processes (e.g. programs targeting frequent hospital admissions and providing these people with additional support, including social services).

- *Local community action programs*—might be centred around community development, but also involve individual and group methods where these are appropriate.
- *Population-level programs*—may use the media and social marketing as an umbrella, but include group and individual processes, capacity building and partnership arrangements as part of community organisation (e.g. the 'Act–Belong-Commit' mental health promotion campaign).

CASE STUDY **9.1**

Detailing success in health promotion

Successes

An analysis of achievements in health promotion from the 1960s to today (a period of rapid growth in chronic diseases) shows that at least half of the more than 30 per cent decline in all cause mortality in Australia has been due to prevention. Most notable are:

- a decrease in male smoking from 75 per cent in 1945 to less than 20 per cent in 2012, resulting in a greater than 20 per cent drop in lung cancer and decreases in heart disease
- a saving of over $8.4 billion from the drop in smoking between 1975 and 1995, which is greater than 50 times that spent on anti-smoking campaigns
- an 80 per cent drop in road trauma deaths from the peak in 1970
- a 75 per cent drop in sudden infant death syndrome (SIDS) since 1980
- a 70 per cent decrease in cyclists killed or with a head injury
- a 30 per cent reduction in mortality due to cancer of the cervix
- a 63 per cent decrease in cardiovascular disease since the peak in 1968
- a decrease in incidence and deaths from AIDS/HIV since its beginnings in 1980.

Lessons

The lessons learned from this have been that good health promotion requires:

1. use of multiple and comprehensive strategies
2. intersectoral collaboration
3. active leadership of the health sector
4. sound epidemiological data informing of the nature and extent of the problem
5. quality research on the effectiveness of interventions and monitoring and surveillance
6. political commitment and clear goals
7. workforce development and training
8. high level and widespread advocacy
9. sustainability of approaches.

Barriers

Barriers needing to be overcome include:

1. lack of leadership on any particular health issue
2. lack of coordination of different levels of government
3. uncontrolled advertising and promotion of competitive, unhealthy products/ services
4. lack of quality information and detailed planning to guide action
5. public apathy or antagonism to change.

NPHT 2009

Selecting strategies

In contemporary societies, many changes occur in social and health behaviour before, and independent of, planned health promotion initiatives. The fitness boom of the 1980s, for example, and the tremendous increases in interest in nutrition and the environment in the 1990s and 2000s, could not realistically be ascribed to any planned health input.

By their very nature of detailed planning and organisation, health promotion activities normally climb onto a wave of public reaction—rather than start that wave. What determines the initial wave is the subject of much scientific speculation, but geopolitic, economic and demographic forces may be as important as any developments in health science.[1]

CASE STUDY **9.2**

Five large-scale prevention studies that have worked

For various reasons, including insufficient resources, inadequate planning and targeting, and the lack of a relevant, guiding conceptual framework, many health promotion interventions have had limited success. On the other hand, there are many successful examples that provide lessons to follow. Some prominent examples include the following:

1. A four-year project in California from 1989–92 used mass media, community-based and school and worksite programs to reduce smoking. There were 33 000 fewer deaths from heart disease in that time than would have been expected based on previous trends (Fichtenberg & Glantz 2000).
2. In Finland, half of a group of 522 middle-aged, overweight men at risk of developing diabetes received individualised counselling about reducing weight, improving diet and increasing physical activity over six years (Uusitupa et al. 2003).

At the end of the trial 58 per cent less of the (lifestyle) intervention group had developed diabetes than the control group (Lindstrom et al. 2003). This and similar studies have been supported by results from a similar intervention where results have persisted for over 20 years in Da Quing, China (Li et al. 2008).

3. In the US a larger study of 3225 men and women at risk of developing diabetes undertook a lifestyle change program (150 minutes physical activity per week plus weight reduction) over four years, compared with a group on a diabetes drug (Metformin) and a control group. Fifty-eight per cent less in the lifestyle group compared to controls progressed to diabetes compared to 33 per cent in the drug group (Knowler et al. 2002).

4. In the Torres Strait (Australia) a diabetes outreach service improved care outcomes for diabetics, but an effective community-based register, managed by local health workers, was critical to its success, reducing diabetes-related hospitalisations by 40 per cent in one year (McDermott et al. 2001).

5. In a sample of schools in the south-west of England, an educational program aimed at reducing the consumption of carbonated soft drinks resulted in a decrease in soft drink intake as well as a significant reduction in weight gain over one year in test schools compared with controls (James et al. 2004).

It is important to remember that although a single specific strategy and/or method may be applicable in a particular circumstance, it is usually necessary to include a number of strategies and methods according to:

- the characteristics of the target group and its needs
- the type of intervention required
- the timeframe of the project
- the goals of the organisation sponsoring the project
- resources available—both financial and human.

What works for one health issue in one place for one period of time may not do so under other circumstances—'*it all depends*'. The skill in health promotion is in analysing and diagnosing—as well as in implementing—the appropriate strategies and methods of intervention. For this reason, to be most effective, the health promotion practitioner should also be familiar with techniques of health promotion planning and program evaluation (covered in Chapter 10).

Strategy selection—individual and population-wide considerations

The traditional focus of health promotion campaigns on individual risk behaviour should be just one part of a comprehensive health promotion program. Australia's National Preventative Health Taskforce (NPHT) sets out a comprehensive strategy approach to tackle tobacco, alcohol and obesity (see Case study 9.3).

CASE STUDY **9.3**

National Preventative Health Taskforce strategy

The National Preventative Health Taskforce (NPHT) was established in 2008 with a mandate to develop a preventive health strategy focusing initially on obesity, tobacco and excessive alcohol consumption. To do this the taskforce identified the following strategic directions:

1. *Shared responsibility*—developing strategic partnerships at all levels of government, industry, business, unions, the non-government sector, research institutions and communities.
2. *Act early and throughout life*—working with individuals, families and communities.
3. *Engage communities*—act and engage with people where they live, work and play at home, in schools, workplaces and the community. Inform, enable and support people to make healthy choices.
4. *Influence markets and develop coherent policies*—for example, through taxation responsive regulation, and through coherent and connected policies.
5. *Reduce inequity through targeting disadvantage*—especially low socioeconomic status population groups.
6. *Indigenous Australians*—contribute to 'Closing the Gap'.
7. *Refocus primary health care* towards prevention.

NPHT 2009

According to new data from the Australian Institute of Health and Welfare (AIHW 2012), it is clear that multiple diseases appear to be linked to homogeneous groups of people. Hence, interventions along the traditional lines of area specialisation may overlook co-existing health problems that have socio-environmental roots. For example, in studies with bus drivers, Syme (1997) noted that this group suffered from high rates of a number of ailments, which may have been simply independent reactions to similar environmental factors—noise, stress and the 'tyranny of the schedule'. 'Upstream' strategies that focus on the total work environment—rather than on individual disease causes—could be more productive and more cost-effective. Therefore, to address the dilemma of the appropriate strategy selection for health promotion, useful advice for the health promotion practitioner has been offered by Hawe and Sheil (1995) who advocated thinking about health promotion programs in the same way as one would conduct a prudent investment portfolio. This would range from 'blue-chip' program investments (evaluated health promotion interventions where the likely impact is either known or more measurable), such as cardiac patient education, through to higher-uncertainty but potentially high-gain investments—such as community capacity building and intersectoral health action.

Garrard et al. (2004) provide a useful example of the issue of strategy selection along the continuum from individual to population level strategies, as applied to cardiovascular disease and diabetes prevention (see Table 9.1).

Table 9.1: CVD–Diabetes Prevention Health Promotion Interventions Framework

Individual focus ←				→ Population focus
Screening, risk factor assessment	Health education Skill development	Social marketing Health information	Community action	Settings and supportive environments
Risk factor assessment and monitoring by general practitioner	Healthy eating/ cooking demonstration Supermarket tours	Local advertising campaign about the benefits of cycling to work	Community reference group to lobby council for safer facilities for physical activity	Collaboration with major workplaces to introduce healthy staff canteen policy
	Education sessions about the benefits of physical activity	'Come and try' day at a local community house	Collaboration with local gym to offer off-peak rates for users	Collaboration with council and workplaces to provide facilities that encourage active transport (such as showers and bike racks)

Garrard et al. 2004

Strategy selection and the diffusion model

In an early approach to dealing with the take-up of a health promotion program, Green and McAlister (1984) made indications about strategy selection based on the diffusion process (introduced in Chapter 2). The basis of this approach is that the adoption of ideas in a community diffuses among individuals in that community at varying rates. Early in the introduction of a new idea or product, 'innovators' and 'early adopters', who are typically more affluent and keyed into national information networks, accept the idea or purchase the product. 'Early' and 'late' majorities are next, and these attend less to national media and more to local media—although they respond less to media in general. The last group to adopt a new idea or product is called 'late adopters', and these people are considered to be the 'hardest to reach' (see Figure 9.1). This diffusion model suggests that different strategies would be more or less effective for targeting the different groups in different phases of the adoption process.

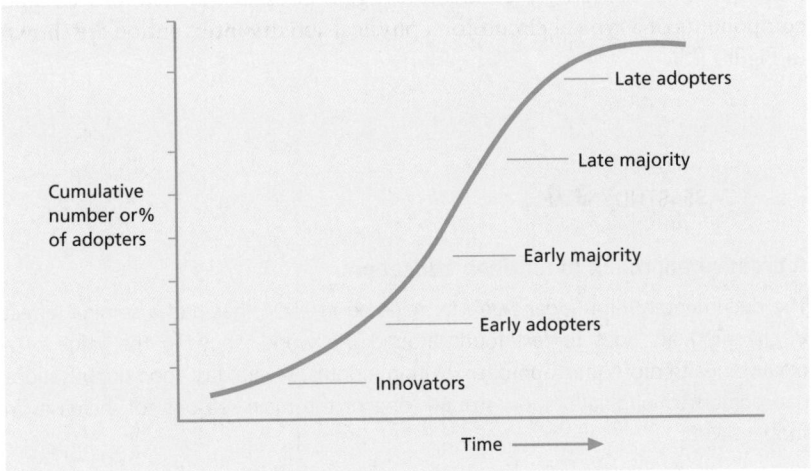

Figure 9.1: **Diffusion of innovation process**

Media may be sufficient for adoption of ideas among innovators and early adopters (i.e. early community leaders who are the social models for the majority), whereas media together with community organisation and capacity-building processes, would be necessary to encourage change in the early and late majority. Community involvement and more intrusive participation programs are necessary to reach late adopters—who are generally, but not always, from disadvantaged groups, with increased health risk.

Strategy selection and needs assessment

A needs assessment in a community is an obvious first start for determining strategy selection. Needs can be assessed at a simple level by observation and situational analysis (see Chapter 10), or more formally through quantitative surveys and epidemiological data collection. There is no hard and fast rule as to how this may be done and different authors provide a variety of different approaches (Gilmore 2011; Green & Kreuter 2004).

One technique developed and used by the current authors is a 'component circuit' approach (Egger, Spark & Donovan 1990). This involves both qualitative and quantitative research (e.g. focus groups, semi-structured interviews, surveys) with a broad range of stakeholders (including end-consumers), in an iterative process, where results from one process feeds forward to the next and then feeds back after modification for verification. This has been used, among other things, to estimate the costs of sports injuries in Australia (Egger 1991) and to develop the Australian National Physical Activity Guidelines (Egger et al. 2001). The process and components of a typical circuit for a physical activity intervention are shown in Figure 9.2.

CASE STUDY **9.4**

A creative approach to nutrition education

The documentary film *Super Size Me*, released in 2004, has had a seminal effect in changing attitudes to fast foods around the world, showing the value of a creative health promotion approach. Within months, several fast food organisations had agreed to eliminate 'super-sizing'—one of the main reasons for increases in food intake.

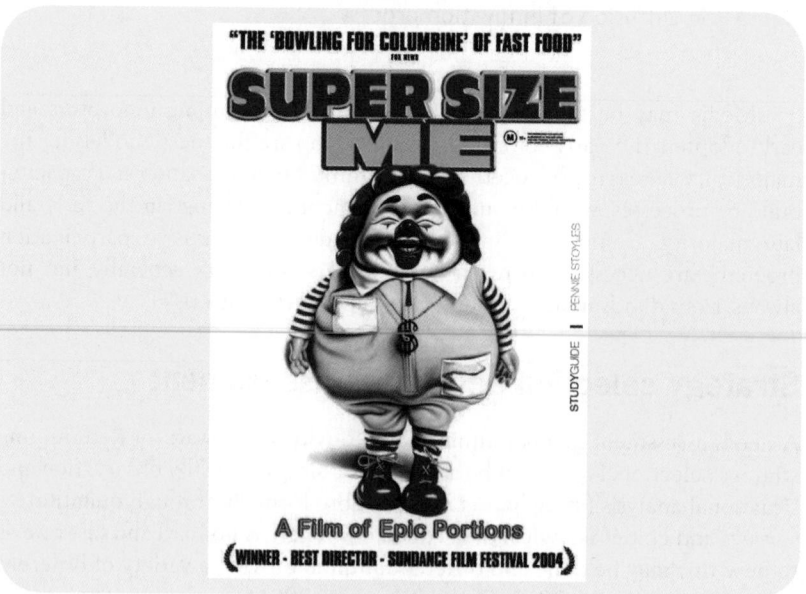

To capitalise on the popularity of the documentary, a study guide became available via the internet for use in schools. This is available at www.imdb.com/title/tt0390521.

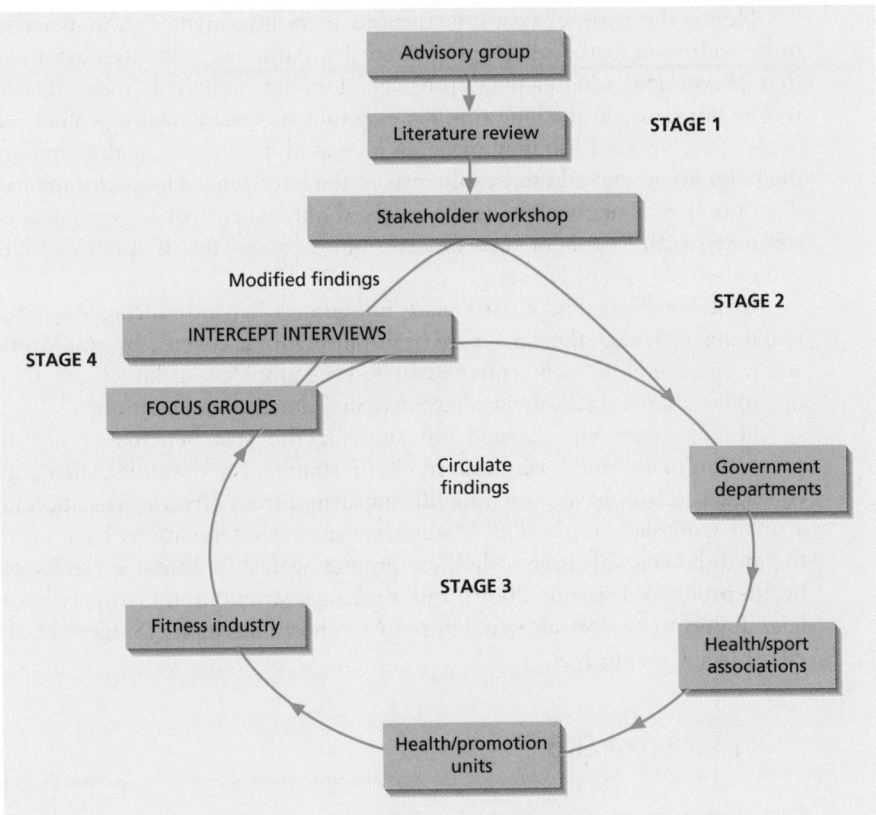

Figure 9.2: Components of a circuit for needs analysis

Strategy selection and costs

In health promotion the days of 'a golden goose laying golden eggs' are long gone—if indeed they ever existed. Sponsoring and funding bodies do not take it on trust that this intervention will reduce health costs in the future. Sponsors now want to see hard data—or at least some outcomes that indicate that programs have been effective in relation to the investment made. Perhaps more than any other professional group, health promotion practitioners can feel vulnerable in the face of calls—frequently from other health professionals— to demonstrate the effectiveness of their programs. In a health system that is increasingly focused on evidence-based methods, health promotion practitioners need, at the very least, to be able to cite some of the evidence that does exist from individually focused interventions, while instruments are developed to evaluate the effectiveness of more complex interventions directed at settings or populations—such as community development interventions.

Hence the issue of cost-effectiveness is an important one that needs to be addressed in the selection of strategies. Although it is often assumed that 'prevention is better than cure', this does not necessarily mean that it will be less costly in the long run. For example, successful health promotion in the early years of life may mean an increased number of aged people in the population who add to health costs in the later years. The philosophical dilemma here is one which can be resolved only when cost-effectiveness is compared with treatment costs in terms of outcome—that is, quality of life and potential years of life saved.

Cost–benefit analysis is particularly important when introducing programs into industry. Unlike the US, where health insurance is covered by employers and where therefore an incentive exists to keep employee-sickness costs to a minimum, there is little obvious incentive in Australian organisations.

Studies have been carried out showing the cost benefits of health promotion in a number of different circumstances. For example, Allen and colleagues (2102) have shown significant savings from lifestyle education in a small workplace in the US; Mediterranean diet interventions have been found to be cost-effective in helping protect against and treat a variety of health problems (Piscopo 2009); and smoking restrictions in Germany have been found to be cost-effective in reducing hospitalisations (Sargent et al. 2012) (see Case study 9.5).

CASE STUDY **9.5**

Cost-effectiveness of health promotion approaches

Health promotion initiatives should be not only shown to work but to be cost-effective in doing so. Data from the Commonwealth Department of Health and Aging show the following cost benefits for different programs.

Tobacco

- Tobacco-control programs in Australia were estimated to have contributed to 10 per cent of the decline in tobacco consumption from 1970 to 1998.
- The estimated net benefit (1970–98) of tobacco control programs was $8.4 billion.

Coronary heart disease

- Public health campaigns were estimated to have contributed to 10 per cent of the reduction in smoking, 30 per cent of the reduction in cholesterol and none of the reduction in blood pressure.

Diabetes

- A cost-effectiveness evaluation indicated that intensive diet/physical activity interventions are more cost-effective than drug treatments ($24 400 and $34 500 respectively per case of diabetes prevented) (DPP 2003).

Cholesterol reduction

- A cost-effectiveness study by Prosser and colleagues in 2000 reported that, overall, diet was substantially more cost-effective than statin therapy for primary prevention of coronary heart disease (CHD) in all 240 risk sub-groups (defined by gender, age and CHD factors) (as cited in Garrard et al. 2004).

Overall

- In the US, a 2008 study showed that for every $1 invested in proven community-based disease prevention programs (increasing physical activity, reducing smoking, improving nutrition), $5.6 (over and above the cost of the program) in savings is returned over the next five years (see http://healthyamericans.org/reports/prevention08).

NPHT 2009

Drug abuse is another area where employers are now appreciating the economies of prevention. Based on US figures, alcoholism in Australian industry could be expected to cost employers around $4 billion per annum, and employer-based programs have been shown to be successful in reducing this cost. There are few data to quantify the increased productivity resulting from increased fitness and wellness of staff but, fortunately, large organisations such as Coles-Myer, Shell, Hewlett-Packard and IBM in Australia have not needed this to develop well-run programs in employee health.

Economic analyses are likely to become of increasing concern as the population ages. Health costs tend to increase for older people who use medical services approximately two to three times as much as those in their middle age. There is therefore an incentive not only for governments but also for health insurance companies (who bear the financial load of supporting this age group) to increase and maintain good health throughout the lifecycle and hence decrease utilisation of services.

Large-scale health promotion programs were criticised in the early days for not showing clear reductions in heart disease death rates (McCormick & Skrahanek 1988). This focus on mortality (rather than quality of life) has led some observers to assume that such interventions were unsuccessful. However, analysis of the data from a number of these programs shows that although *mortality* was not affected, there was a significant 'compression of morbidity' in older people, resulting in less need for health services in the later years. This has also been found to be the case with the large scale Look AHEAD study in the US. Mortality rates from preventive interventions for diabetes reduction in this trial have not been reduced, but other health and fitness indices have improved (Jakicic et al. 2012). If quality of life is improved in the later years, *active* life expectancy—that is, those years in which disease is relatively absent—is extended. Evidence that supports this contention is also emerging from research indicating that

231

high-intensity strength-training exercises are an effective and feasible means to preserve bone density while improving muscle mass, strength and balance in older people (Hunter, McCarthy & Bammam 2004). This information is useful for developing policy aiming health promotion services at older adults.

CASE STUDY **9.6**

Lessons learned from the tobacco experience for obesity control

The fight against smoking, which began with evidence of the adverse effects of smoking in the 1950s and was translated in earnest into anti-smoking programs in the early 1970s, provides a number of lessons in changing population health. There are similar social, psychological and environmental factors between this and the modern obesity epidemic, suggesting that the key elements of an obesity-control program should include (1) clinical intervention and management—with physicians being an effective way of doing this; (2) educational strategies, both at the individual and population levels; (3) regulatory efforts, such as control over the number and nature of food outlets in vulnerable areas, such as schools; (4) economic approaches, through taxing and incentive schemes; and (5) the combination of all of these into comprehensive programs that address multiple facets of the environment simultaneously.

Mercer et al. 2003

In the final two chapters we put all of the information from the preceding chapters together to look at a process for planning health promotion interventions, and some useful skills and tools for the practitioner.

Note

1. For a discussion of how these social movements or changes develop, see *The Tipping Point* by Malcolm Gladwell, 2002, Back Bay Books, New York.

References

AIHW (Australian Institute of Health and Welfare), 2012, Multiple causes of death, *Bulletin 105*;Aug, AIHW, Canberra.

Allen, J.C., Lewis, J.B., & Tagliaferro, A.R., 2012, Cost-effectiveness of health risk reduction after lifestyle education in the small workplace, *Prev Chronic Dis* 9:E96. Epub May 10.

DPP (Diabetes Prevention Program), 2003, Costs associated with the primary prevention of type 2 diabetes mellitus in the Diabetes Prevention Program, *Diabetes Care* 26(1):36–47.

Egger, G., 1991, Sports injuries in Australia: causes, costs and prevention, *Health Promot J Aust* 1(2): 28–33.

Egger, G., Donovan, R., Giles-Corti, B., Bull, F., & Swinburn, B., 2001, Developing national physical activity guidelines for Australians, *Aust NZ J Public Health* 25(6):561–3.

Egger, G., Spark, R., & Donovan, R.A, 1990, 'Component circuit analysis' to needs assessment and strategy selection in health promotion, *Health Promot Int* 5(4):299–302.

Fichtenberg, C.M., & Glantz, S.A., 2000, Association of the California Tobaccco Control Program with declines in cigarette consumption and mortality from heart disease, *New Engl J Med* 343(24):1772–7.

Garrard, J., Lewis, B., Keleher, H., Tunny, N., Burke L., Harper, S. & Round R., 2004, *Planning for Healthy Communities: Reducing the Risk of Cardiovascular Disease and Type 2 Diabetes through Healthier Environments and Lifestyles*, Victorian Government Department of Human Services, Melbourne.

Gilmore, G., 2011, *Needs and Capacity Assessment Strategies for Health Education and Health Promotion* (3rd edn), Jones and Bartlett, Sudbury, Massachusetts.

Green, L.W., & Kreuter M.W., 2004, *Health Promotion Planning: An Ecological Approach*, Jones and Bartlett, Sudbury, Massachusetts.

Green, L.W., & McAlister, A.L., 1984, Macro-intervention to support health behaviour: some theoretical perspectives and practical reflections, *Health Educ Quarterly* 11(3):332–9.

Hawe, P., & Sheil, A., 1995, Preserving innovation under increasing accountability pressures: the health promotion investment portfolio approach, *Health Promot J Aust* 5(2):4–9.

Hunter, G.R., McCarthy, J.P., & Bamman M.M., 2004, Effects of resistance training on older adults, *Sports Med* 34(5):329–48.

Jakicic, J.M., Egan, C.M., Fabricatore, A.N., Gaussoin, S.A., Glasser, S.P., Hesson, L.A., Knowler, W.C., Lang, W., Regensteiner, J.G., Ribisl, P.M., & Ryan, D.H., 2012, The Look AHEAD Research Group, 2012, Four-year change in cardiorespiratory fitness and influence on glycemic control in adults with type 2 diabetes in a randomized trial: the Look AHEAD Trial, *Diabetes Care* 6 Dec [Epub ahead of print].

James, J., Thomas, P., Cavan, D., & Kerr, D., 2004, Preventing childhood obesity by reducing consumption of carbonated drinks: cluster randomised controlled trial, *BMJ* 328:1237–9.

Knowler, W.C., Barrett-Connor, E., Fowler, S.E., Hammman, R.F., Lachan, J.M., Walker, E.A., & Natahn, D.M., 2002, Diabetes Prevention Research Group. Reduction in the incidence of type 2 diabetes with lifestyle intervention or metformin, *N Engl J Med* 346:393–403

Li, G., Wang, J., Gregg, EQ., et al., 2008, The long-term effect of lifestyle interventions to prevent diabetes in the China Da Qing Diabetes Prevention Study: a 20-year follow-up study, *Lancet* 371(9626):1783–9.

Lindstrom, J., Louheranta, A., Mannelin, M., Rastas, M., Salminen, V., Eriksson, J., Uusitupa, M., & Tuomilehto, J. and for the Finnish Diabetes Prevention Study Group, 2003. The Finnish Diabetes Prevention Study (DPS): lifestyle intervention and 3-year results on diet and physical activity, *Diabetes Care* Dec;26(12):3230–6.

McCormick, J., & Skrahanek, P., 1988, Coronary heart disease is not preventable by population interventions, *Lancet* II:839–41.

McDermott, R., Tulip, F., Schmidt B., & Sinha, A., 2001, Sustaining better diabetes care in remote indigenous Australian communities, *BMJ* 327:428–30.

Mercer, S.L., Green, L.W., Rosenthal, A.C., Husten, C.G., Khan, L.K., & Dietz, W.H., 2003, Possible lessons from the tobacco experience for obesity control, *Am J Clin Nutr* 77(4 Suppl):1073S–82S.

NPHT (National Preventative Health Taskforce), 2009, *Australia: The Healthiest Country by 2020. National Preventative Health Strategy—Overview*, NPHT, Canberra.

Piscopo, S., 2009, The Mediterranean diet as a nutrition education, health promotion and disease prevention tool, *Public Health Nutr* 12(9A):1648–55.

Sargent, J.D., Demidenko, E., Malenka, D.J., Gohlke, H., & Hanewinkel, R., 2012, Smoking restrictions and hospitalization for acute coronary events in Germany, *Clin Res Cardiol* 101(3):227–35.

Spark, R., Donovan, R J., & Howat, P., 1991, Promoting health and preventing injury in remote Aboriginal communities: a case study, *Health Promot J Aust* 1(2):10–16.

Syme, L.S., 1997, Individual vs community interventions in public health practice: some thoughts about a new approach, *Health Promot Matters (VicHealth)* 2:2–9.

Uusitupa M., Lindi V., Louheranta A., Salopuro T., Lindstrom J., & Tuomilehto J., 2003, Long-term improvement in insulin sensitivity by changing lifestyles of people with impaired glucose tolerance: 4-year results from the Finnish diabetes prevention study, *Diabetes* 52(1):2532–8.

chapter 10

Putting it all together: planning health promotion initiatives

Summary of main points

- There are a number of different planning models for implementing health promotion.
- The tested PRECEDE–PROCEDE model identifies key factors in any program and helps structure a program from the outset.
- Transition models such as SOPIE provide a graduated, phased approach to putting a program into action.
- All appropriate approaches involve planning, implementation and evaluation.

Program planning

In this chapter we attempt to bring together the practical aspects of designing an integrated health promotion program as discussed in the preceding chapters. This involves applying general principles of planning to the identification of needs, and developing strategies and methods to meet these needs. The development of any program—regardless of the specific planning approach—will depend on a range of factors, such as the nature of the topic to be addressed, the size of the intended target group or population group, involvement of local stakeholders, the skills and abilities of the health promotion specialist, and the desires of the target community. Planning a pool fencing campaign for a local government area in a New Zealand city, for example, would require a different perspective to planning an obesity reduction campaign for a Pacific Island country, although the planning conceptual framework may be the same in each case. Hence the planning framework selected must be sufficiently comprehensive and flexible to accommodate a wide variety of health promotion strategies and methods.

A number of planning models have been described, all of which include valuable planning constructs. Some are based around strategies for different phases of the lifespan (Edelman, Mandel & Edelman 2002; Murray & Zentnor 2001), while others are specifically settings-based such as within workplaces (e.g. Cox 2003) or in clinical practice (Woolf, Jonas & Lawrence 1996). Perhaps the simplest distillation of a planning process is that shown in Figure 10.1, modified from one of the most widely accepted exponents in this area—Lawrence Green (Green & Kreuter 1999).

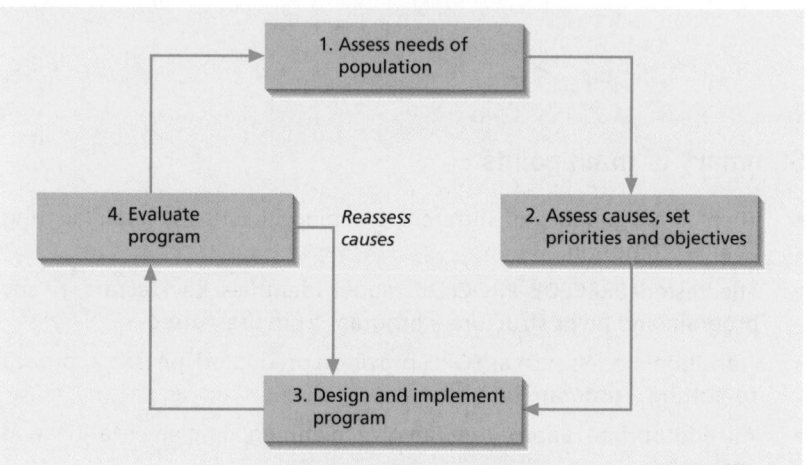

Figure 10.1: **Green's basic steps in program planning and implementation**
Green & Kreuter 1999

In this model, phase 1 implies an epidemiological approach to identifying populations at risk and determining needs overall. In phase 2, risk factors are identified, both behavioural (e.g. alcohol, tobacco, physical inactivity, diet, unsafe driving behaviours) and structural (e.g. poor housing, unemployment, unsafe work environments), along with Green's predisposing, enabling and reinforcing factors (Green & Kreuter 2005) (see below). Phase 3 involves the design and implementation of a program to deal with this, and phase 4 looks at evaluation and re-assessment of the program.

The PRECEDE–PROCEED model

The PRECEDE–PROCEED model is probably the most widely used planning model in the health promotion literature and in practice. A survey of members of the Australian Health Promotion Association in 2004 found that the PRECEDE–PROCEED was the model most frequently used for program planning and implementation (Jones & Donovan 2004), and Green's website lists well over 1000 publications referring to the model, with most of them involving an application of the model. Applications range from the usual areas of tobacco, nutrition, physical activity, sun protection, road safety and alcohol, to occupational health, domestic violence, periodontal treatment and juvenile rheumatoid arthritis—and even how to get university professors to be more productive (i.e. 'Using the PRECEDE–PROCEED model to increase productivity in health education faculty', Ransdell 2001).

The PRECEDE–PROCEED model has been applied in a variety of countries, including India, Nepal, Taiwan, France, the Netherlands, Australia, Canada, France and Spain, and among various ethnic sub-groupings in the US and Canada (Donovan & Henley 2010; see www.lgreen.net/precede. htm, which includes a version of the model in Japanese). The model is shown in Figure 10.2 and the use of the model to develop a mental health intervention is shown in Figure 10.3 (from Wright et al. 2006).

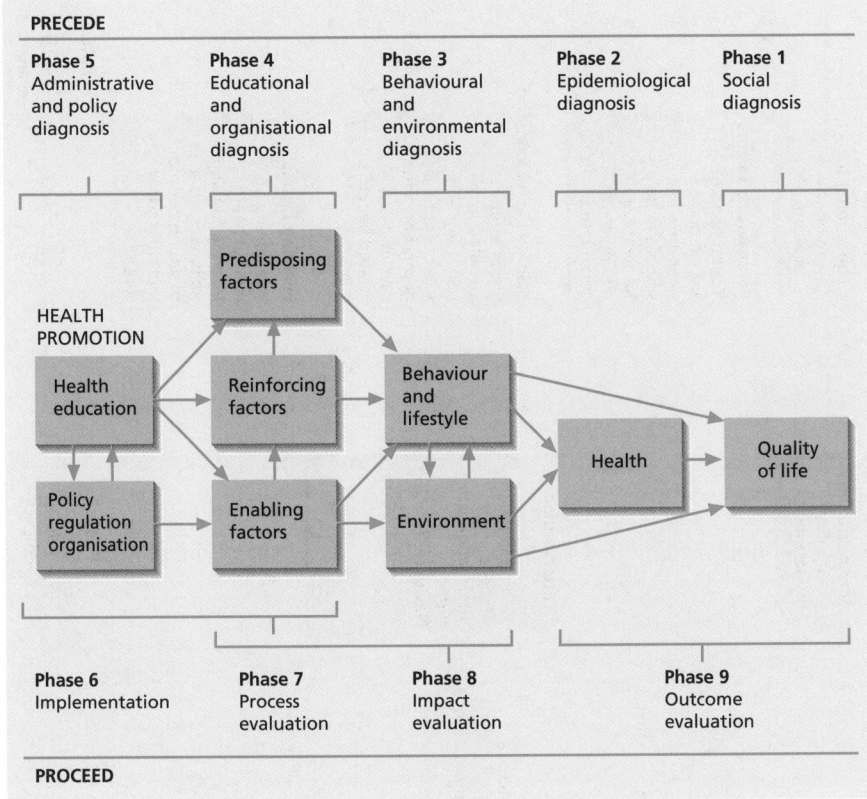

Figure 10.2: The PRECEDE–PROCEED model for health promotion planning and evaluation

Green & Kreuter 2005

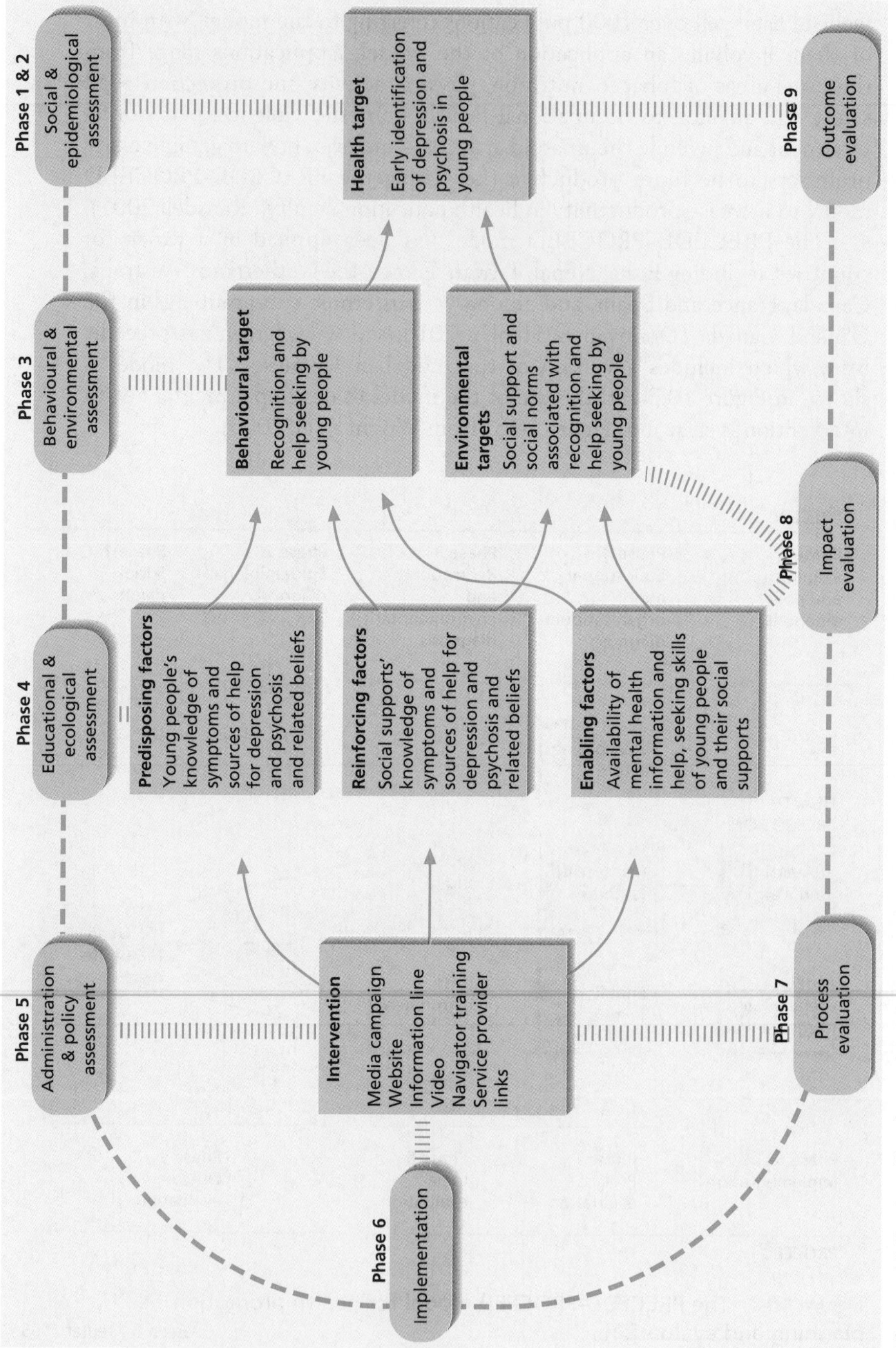

Figure 10.3: Application of PRECEDE–PROCEED to a mental health intervention

© 2006 Wright et al.; licensee BioMed Central Ltd

Phase 1 & 2
Social & epidemiological assessment

Health target
Early identification of depression and psychosis in young people

Phase 3
Behavioural & environmental assessment

Behavioural target
Recognition and help seeking by young people

Environmental targets
Social support and social norms associated with recognition and help seeking by young people

Phase 4
Educational & ecological assessment

Predisposing factors
Young people's knowledge of symptoms and sources of help for depression and psychosis and related beliefs

Reinforcing factors
Social supports' knowledge of symptoms and sources of help for depression and psychosis and related beliefs

Enabling factors
Availability of mental health information and help, seeking skills of young people and their social supports

Phase 5
Administration & policy assessment

Intervention
Media campaign
Website
Information line
Video
Navigator training
Service provider links

Phase 6
Implementation

Phase 7
Process evaluation

Phase 8
Impact evaluation

Phase 9
Outcome evaluation

The value of Green's model (which has undergone a number of modifications since first presented as just PRECEDE) is that it makes explicit that the factors analysed in the planning and development phases (the PRECEDE phases) are the same factors to be considered in the implementation and evaluation phases (PROCEED).

PRECEDE is an acronym for Predisposing, Reinforcing and Enabling Constructs in Educational (and Environmental) Diagnosis and Evaluation. According to Spark (1999), who applied the model to his PhD thesis on health promotion in Indigenous communities, the PRECEDE framework was novel in that it focused on outcomes rather than inputs, forcing the health practitioner to begin the planning process from the outcome end. It was also comprehensive in that each of the original five phases in PRECEDE allows a different 'layer' of assessment: social, epidemiological, behavioural, educational and administrative.

During the decade following the publication of PRECEDE, there was an acknowledgment in the international public health community that health education, with its emphasis on behavioural or lifestyle-related choices and individually oriented programmes, was neglecting the importance of social factors in the aetiology of many diseases.

Responding to this neglect, Green amended the PRECEDE model to give greater emphasis to environmental factors and expanded it to include PROCEED, an acronym for Policy, Regulatory and Organisational Constructs in Educational and Environmental Development. PROCEED includes resource mobilisation and evaluation and is essentially an elaboration and extension of the original administrative diagnosis phase of PRECEDE. Overall, the addition of PROCEED to the original model gave greater emphasis to the contribution of structural factors and community organisation processes to program implementation.

Donovan and Henley (2010) provide the following outline of the PRECEDE–PROCEED model and its application. The phase 1 social assessment involves assessing people's perceptions of their own needs and how the issue at hand impacts on their quality of life. For example, people with asthma and diabetes face certain restrictions on their lifestyle, have to comply with a medication schedule and have to visit a medical practitioner more often than average. Epidemiological analyses (phase 2) identify the relative importance of various health problems in various sub-groups of the population, and the behavioural and environmental factors related to those health problems. For example, young males account for a higher proportion of road crashes than other groups; alcohol, speed, fatigue and not wearing a seat belt are related to crashes, severity of injury and mortality.

Behavioural and environmental analyses look at the factors arising from epidemiological analyses in more depth, as well as behaviours and

239

environmental aspects that may arise from clinical or other evidence. In road safety, the use of seat belts, driver education, driver skills, exceeding the speed limit, driving while tired, vehicular modifications, roadworthiness of vehicles, road conditions and placement of warning signs all require analysis in terms of such things as how important they are, how changeable they are and what resources are required to change them.

Phase 3, the educational and ecological assessment, is the 'core' of the model: it identifies the factors that must be changed to initiate or facilitate the desired behaviour and environmental changes. These factors then become the targets for the program. The model proposes three types of factors:

- *Predisposing factors*—individuals' beliefs, attitudes and perceptions that influence their decision to act (e.g. a belief that alcohol increases feelings of wellbeing and reduces one's shyness predisposes one to consume alcohol; a belief that alcohol is a poison or may lead to loss of control predisposes one to not consume alcohol).
- *Reinforcing factors*—environmental factors that serve to reward or punish expression of the behaviour (e.g. friends' approval of one's speeding or drinking alcohol serves to reinforce the behaviour; a moral stance against drug use serves to inhibit that behaviour).
- *Enabling factors*—individual and environmental factors that make a behaviour possible (or not possible) to occur (e.g. having time and money facilitates joining a health club; smokefree policies facilitate smoking cessation in terms of skills, resources, support policies and services).

For example, following research with regard to drink driving among male drivers in rural areas, Batini and Donovan (2001) proposed the classification of factors influencing drink driving in the following areas.

Predisposing factors

- *Convenience*—most believe that it's simply easier to drive rather than seek out alternatives. They believe it's easier to drive home than collect their car the next day (includes fear of damage to or theft of car if left overnight).
- *Cultural acceptance*—rather than being 'morally unacceptable' behaviour, drinking and driving is very much seen as being 'culturally acceptable'—the actual social norm in their towns. However, they do distinguish between the terms 'drinking and driving' versus 'drunk driving', the latter being generally considered far less 'acceptable'.
- *Personal safety*—in some towns many were fearful of being assaulted while walking home after having consumed alcohol.

Enabling factors

- *Lack of enforcement*—most participants knew that 'the police can't be everywhere all the time'. Many knew the time when the police 'knocked off' for the evening. High profile 'blitzes' (e.g. booze bus, random breath test stop) are highly visible and easily avoided (via the 'bush telegraph). There was a known lack of funding for regular patrols and a perception that if they have got away with it before, they can get away with it again.
- *Lack of public transport*—for many, there are simply no (or very limited) public transport options, particularly within the smaller towns. In addition, those living out of town cite the distance as being too far to walk (e.g. 30 km, 50 km).

Reinforcing factors

- *Expense of alternatives*—many are reluctant to pay the fare for a 30–50-kilometre taxi ride—often viewed as a 'waste of good drinking money'.
- *Confidence*—while aware of the 0.05 blood alcohol limit, many feel perfectly capable of driving above this limit, citing that they've 'driven from an early age on the farm' and have the 'ability to handle country roads'. Others try to drive more 'carefully' after drinking (e.g. slower, concentrate more). There is a perception that if they have been able to successfully drive home after consuming alcohol before, they can do it again.

The educational and organisational analysis identifies what needs to be done. The next phase looks at how it can be done. Administrative and policy assessment involves assessing resources and looking at educational, motivational and regulatory alternatives for influencing the factors identified in phase 4. It involves establishing intersectoral collaboration where necessary and developing relationships with intermediaries.

Planning and designing the intervention are an outcome of phases 1–4, along with setting of process, impact and outcome objectives. Implementation (phase 5) can include pre-testing of methods and materials, perhaps even carrying out efficacy (or pilot) trials of the intervention. Process evaluation should be ongoing to ensure that timelines are met and to enable valid assessments of impact and outcomes (e.g. failure to meet attitudinal and behavioural objectives might be due to non-delivery of communication materials; call analyses might reveal that only 20 per cent of calls to a helpline are being answered before the caller hangs up).

CASE STUDY **10.1**

Applying PRECEDE–PROCEED to increasing fruit and vegetable consumption

For the US Black Churches United for Better Health Project, Campbell et al. (1999) used the PRECEDE–PROCEED model to develop a set of activities based on the predisposing, enabling and reinforcing factors identified as determinants of fruit and vegetable consumption.

They reported the following activities to address predisposing factors:

- *Tailored bulletins*—each individual received personalised, tailored messages and feedback based on questionnaire data with regard to their beliefs, attitudes and current behaviours, barriers, social support and stage of change.
- *Printed materials*—monthly packages of brochures, posters, banners, idea sheets, church bulletin inserts were provided to each church's nutrition action team (church members recruited by the pastor to organise and implement activities).

The following activities addressed enabling factors:

- *Gardening*—churches were encouraged to plant fruit and vegetable gardens and training was available for 'master gardeners'. (Note: A program in Queensland encouraged schools to plant gardens as a way of creating and sustaining positive attitudes towards fruit and vegetable consumption—see Viola 2002.)
- *Educational sessions*—Nutrition action team members attended educational sessions and were trained to conduct cooking sessions showing how to achieve 'five a day' guidelines.
- *Cookbook and recipe tasting*—a trained 'cookbook person' in each church showed members how to modify their favourite recipes to meet the 'five a day' guidelines and conducted taste tests on the modified products. Recipes were included in a cookbook distributed to all participants.
- *Serving more fruit and vegetables at church functions*—a 'practise what you preach' orientation to enable more trial of fruit and vegetable dishes.

The following activities addressed reinforcing factors:

- *Lay health advisors*—identified 'natural helpers' were identified and trained on social support to assisting others advance through the stages of change.
- *Community coalitions*—each county formed a coalition of relevant stakeholders such as local grocers, farmers and church members who received training in community action and organised community events.
- *Pastor support*—pastors were encouraged to promote the campaign in their sermons and church announcements, received a newsletter keeping them informed of all activities, reviewed educational materials and were involved in generating tailored messages.

- *Grocer-vendor involvement*—promotional materials such as recipe cards, coupons and farmer's market posters were distributed to church members and local stores.

Donovan & Henley 2010

SOPIE—a model for planning and initiating health promotion

An alternative five stage planning model used by the authors has the acronym SOPIE. The five stages are:

- Situational analysis
- Objective setting
- Planning
- Implementation
- Evaluation

The SOPIE approach has been used in Pacific Island countries to help structure interventions aimed at reducing chronic, non-communicable diseases such as diabetes and obesity, as well as in smaller scale social experiments such as in encouraging older people to eat more fibre. The stages are discussed in detail below and summarised in the box.

The SOPIE model for health promotion interventions

- **S**ituational analysis—identifying the issue, specifying the problem, identifying potential target audiences and strategies, assessing resources, formative research
- **O**bjective setting—defining overall goals, campaign goals and specific behavioural and communication objectives for the target audiences
- **P**lanning—devising message and intervention strategies, developing and pre-testing materials, selecting media, identifying supporting components
- **I**mplementation—developing detailed program procedures, involvement of other sectors and stakeholders, program management
- **E**valuation—campaign monitoring, process and outcome evaluation

---

Stage 1: Situational analysis

This stage is intended to identify and accurately represent the extent of the problem or issue and to identify possible causes. It is perhaps the most important stage of any campaign and that for which most input is necessary.

There are four distinct phases within this: identifying the problems, defining the intended target group or population, identifying possible strategies and generating a strategic concept.

Identifying the problem

Problem identification can come from a number of sources including literature reviews, epidemiological data, political interest, statistics, a formal needs analysis or public pressure. While there may be a need based on the frequency and severity of the problem, social (and political) attitudes can influence the process of priority setting. Public acceptance of both the problem and the solution are important ingredients for successful intervention. The practical elements of analysis therefore include:

1. the nature and extent of the problem (e.g. frequency, severity)
2. the level of evidence relating to the proposed problem (e.g. will decreasing smoking consumption actually reduce lung cancer?)
3. public and political acceptance for (a) an action to be taken and (b) the proposed action to be taken (e.g. would the public accept, and would politicians pay for, a major campaign based on quitting smoking?).

It should be noted that often the problem is not as it initially seems. Early campaigns aimed at reducing smoking, for example, were based on increasing knowledge of the health risks of smoking. As these results became known, it was clearer that the problem was not so much knowledge, but building feelings of being able to quit, and facilitating quitting by increasing social pressure to quit.

Defining the intended target group or population

Once a problem is identified, there is a need to clearly identify the intended target group or population. This is not necessarily those for whom the problem is greatest. It might be those who are most likely to be influenced, given the available resources (i.e. where the health promoter is likely to get the best return on investment).

Smokers, for example, can be segmented on a number of factors such as age, gender, length of time smoking, acceptance of health messages or willingness to quit. A segment selected for a quit smoking program may not necessarily be the largest (e.g. young women), but could be smokers with the most to gain from quitting and may be likely to have contemplated doing so (e.g. pregnant women), or those who are the easiest to reach given limited resources.

Identifying possible strategies

In this stage of planning, the viability of using complementary strategies as outlined throughout this text is assessed, and the role each is to play vis-a-vis other strategies is determined. Furthermore, any comprehensive program must consider and select *all* strategies that can add to the aims of the program. This could include changes in availability of products or materials (e.g. higher taxes on energy-dense foods leading to obesity, restriction of fast food outlets) and changes in conditions encouraging overeating (e.g. improvements in school canteens), as well as capacity building among community-based groups to help progression towards the program goal. As suggested by the epidemiological triad considered in Chapter 1, it is only when *all* corners of the triad are considered that an epidemic (or health problem) can be truly managed.

Generating a strategic concept

Where appropriate, ideas for a project concept or major theme are often developed at this stage using either formative research or skilled assessment by health professionals. A strategic concept is a broad approach to the issue at hand that provides direction for the definition of communication objectives and the development of program strategies. For instance, in the case of skin cancer prevention, a concept may be to encourage greater use of shaded environments. This might then lead to a strategy of either working with local communities and authorities to provide more shade or developing a media campaign to encourage individuals to seek out existing shade options.

Summary of tasks in stage 1

Main tasks
- Identify and describe the problem.
- Identify and describe target groups.
- Identify strategies to reach and impact the target groups.
- Generate an overall strategic concept or theme for the campaign.

Stage 2: Objective setting

Based on the identified problem and the selection of intended audiences, the next step is to set overall goals and specific behavioural and communication objectives for the intended audience(s).

Defining goals

Goals help to determine the direction of an intervention and set forth what the program hopes to achieve. Goals are written as broad general statements. An example to do with sexually transmitted infections may be 'to decrease infertility in women due to sexually transmitted infections'.

Because they are broad and general, goals need to be accompanied by specific measurable objectives.

Setting objectives

The planning stage of any project is designed to provide a blueprint for action. As part of this, there is a need for a set of clear-cut objectives determined with the local community. Ideally, the objectives of a well-planned campaign should be specific, time related and measurable. They can be defined in terms of the ultimately desired outcome (e.g. reduced morbidity) or intermediate objectives such as target population knowledge, attitudes and behaviours; changes in the physical environment; or public policy or practices related to health. In the case of motor vehicle injuries, the overall objective of a preventive initiative may be reduced fatalities, but intermediate measures such as a reduction in driver blood alcohol levels, or even reduction of alcohol consumption in a targeted area, could be included as intermediate objectives.

Project objectives must be realistic. What can be achieved by one, limited-duration campaign must not be confused with what is hoped could be achieved by a series of campaigns and a combination of strategies that would be part of a long-term program.

Capacity building, stakeholder involvement and environmental diagnosis

This stage can include capacity building, particularly where this is likely to be important for later healthcare worker involvement. In the case of type 2 diabetes prevention, for example, training in management of obesity and weight control for clinicians might be a vital component of any program. This can also help to ensure greater cooperation of medical and other health professionals in ongoing program development. Capacity building of healthcare workers in the basic principles of health promotion can also be included here.

Because any initiatives must be developed and 'owned' by the community in which they are to be enacted, key stakeholders need to be incorporated into any planning decisions. One way of doing this is by involving these people in an environmental analysis such as using the ANGELO model (see Chapter 8, p. 194), which then serves the dual function of increasing community involvement as well as helping the community define its own issues.

Summary of tasks in stage 2

Main tasks

- Build community links.
- Build baseline capacity building (e.g. medical and allied health professional education).
- Environmental diagnosis (e.g. ANGELO) and stakeholder involvement.
- Enhance health promotion capacity (e.g. by workshops with local health promotion staff).
- Set potential goals and objectives with health personnel.

Stage 3: Planning

Once detailed objectives have been set, the next step is to develop specific project components. The viability and affordability of different potential strategies needs to be assessed; message strategies and the media for their dissemination need to be identified; monitoring and evaluation procedures should be specified; pre-testing undertaken where necessary; and other back-up strategies devised. The role of other sectors needs to be defined and their cooperation sought. Adequate resources must be available to meet the anticipated response to the campaign (e.g. domestic violence campaigns inevitably result in a large number of abused persons seeking counselling).

Choosing the method

Once strategies have been devised, the methods of operation need to be considered. If population-wide awareness raising is an option, different approaches to delivering the message should be considered. As stated in Chapter 6, mass media advertising is expensive, but allows full control over message exposure and greater flexibility in presentation; publicity is relatively inexpensive, but depends to a great extent on the 'newsworthiness' of a topic; and edutainment is even less able to be controlled by the message initiator and is likely only to work over the long term. Choice of method also depends on the target group or population, the project objectives and the budget, as well as the availability of appropriate skills to the health team.

Where a community process is selected as an appropriate strategy, methods of involving the community such as through social mobilisation, leader or skill group meetings, or partnership arrangements may need to be considered.

Developing the message/s

Message development involves first *getting the right message*, and second *getting the message right* so that it is delivered in a way likely to be most effective. Given a behavioural or attitudinal objective, *getting the right message* attempts to answer the question: what sort of motivations must be aroused or what sort of beliefs need to be established in the receivers' minds to bring about these behavioural or attitudinal changes? The primary tools for message strategy development are qualitative research techniques such as individual indepth interviews and focus group discussions with members of the target audience.

The message strategy should include the following elements, although not always in every individual message execution:

1. the benefits promised by adopting the recommended behaviour or attitude (i.e. the motivational component)
2. specific actions that the individual, or community can undertake, whether intermediate (e.g. call a hotline) or related to the desired end behaviour

3. reassurances that the recommended course of action is efficacious
4. reassurances that the individual or community is capable of carrying out the recommended course of action (with appropriate assistance where relevant).

Where more than one strategy is used, which usually should be the case, the relative roles of the strategies and methods within these need to be established and the subsequent activities for each method developed with these different objectives in mind.

Testing the message/s

Before full-scale implementation of a project, communication materials should be pre-tested. This can include such processes as concept testing and efficacy testing (Donovan & Henley 2010). Pre-testing messages at this stage can provide direction for improving the message or identifying which of several alternative strategies for execution has the greatest potential. A number of communication models are available for this stage of the planning, including the Centre for Disease Control's CDCynergy DVD tools (www.cdc.gov/healthcommunication/CDCynergy) (see also Donovan & Henley 2010).

Summary of tasks in stage 3

Main tasks
- Plan an ongoing and sustainable project.
- Link allied groups.
- Provide further education (e.g. of medical and health professionals) where appropriate.
- Consider evaluation methods and baseline evaluation research.
- Plan an awareness-raising 'umbrella' where appropriate and possible.
- Develop communication materials.
- Select main messages and methods of delivery.

Stage 4: Implementation

Implementing a health promotion program includes setting process objectives (i.e. what is to be accomplished, by whom and when), managing the implementation process (i.e. coordination, intersectoral liaison), monitoring the process and being prepared for any negative responses to the campaign.

Process objectives detail the level of activities designed to produce the desired outcomes. Process objectives are not simply lists of activities but are quantifiable and measurable statements of what the project will have accomplished by certain dates. For reducing motor vehicle injuries, for example, process objectives could include the number of community service announcements to be aired by a certain date, the number of media releases to have been issued by that date, the number of roadside breath tests conducted, the number of speed cameras operating for certain periods of time, and what proportion of the target population becomes aware of the campaign and its relevance to them.

Some projects involve a staged 'rollout' of strategies. The first stage of an alcohol implementation, for example, may concentrate on increasing knowledge of less well known risks (e.g. alcohol and increased risk of various cancers). A second and later stage may be advocacy orientated, aimed at increasing pressure on politicians to introduce greater restrictions on opening hours, low-cost promotions and outlet density. Health promotion projects using the media in 'new' topic areas, where knowledge and awareness is low, often aim initially at educating (or informing) about the problem, then run a second stage to motivate (or persuade) the target audiences to do something about this.

Monitoring is important in the implementation stage to ensure that activities are being implemented as planned, that appropriate changes are occurring and to evaluate the process of operation. This is often done through a recording of requests received about a program or other tracking measures. Enquiries for further information, increased demand for project materials or courses, or increases in the sales of appropriate products (e.g. fruits and vegetables, exercise equipment, nicotine chewing gum, gym memberships) may be relevant measures of whether the message is reaching and impacting its target audience.

It should also be recognised that often there are vested interests opposed to project methods that seek to alter the status quo, and reaction from these is likely to come at or even prior to the implementation stage of any campaign. Alcohol marketers, for example, form a powerful lobby group against measures designed to reduce alcohol sponsorship of sport as a means of reducing alcohol consumption among young people, and food and beverage manufacturers will try to counter any attempts to reduce the sale of certain foods and soft drinks.

If possible, these contingencies should be forecast in the planning stages and approaches developed for coping with them as they arise. In some cases, interference in a health promotion project has been used by health professionals to create publicity around a promotion, which ensures that it achieves a wider exposure than might otherwise have occurred.

In this phase, demand should be anticipated for the increased need for 'on the ground' services. A quit smoking project, for example, might increase the need for quit smoking courses, self-help groups and nicotine patches and gums; diabetes prevention may stimulate an interest in weight control and exercise programs; and traffic injury prevention may require driver training skills. These needs should be anticipated in the early stage of the project to ensure adequate resource allocation and the continuation of momentum of the project once this has begun.

Summary of tasks in stage 4

Main tasks
- Put the plan into action.
- Involve the community and relevant stakeholders.
- Establish 'on-the-ground' services (e.g. quit smoking groups, weight loss education centres, etc); ongoing capacity building of health professionals.
- Develop advocacy skills to counter anticipated—and unanticipated— opposition from vested interests in particular.

Garrard et al. (2004) from Deakin University provide an excellent example of a summary planning grid for a hypothetical health promotion program ('Healthy People, Healthy Places') in a fictitious community (Banksia Bay) in the document *Planning for Healthy Communities* (www. health.vic.gov.au/healthpromotion/downloads/healthy_communities.pdf) (see Case study 10.2).

CASE STUDY **10.2**

Planning grid for a health promotion program

Health promotion interventions and capacity-building strategies	Estimated reach	Timelines and by whom	Estimated budget	OPTIONAL Estimated other funding sources
Community action A 'walkability' audit by community groups of their local areas feedback to a council action group OR	Specific groups, such as women with young children, older women, non-English speaking income groups	Project facilitator coordinate feedback (dates)	Photocopying and mailout audit tool	Rotary and other clubs

A community event such as 'Ride to work day'				
Settings and supportive environments Intersectorial partnership to increase the percentage of workplaces with policies to improve facilities (e.g. showers, bike parking, the use of bicycles)	Management and employees at the workplace	Agency Management Local government staff/ management		
Organisational development Collaborative, interdisciplinary working group (coordinated by the local government area) to address issues for safe cycling and walking	The population in general will benefit from improved environments for active transport	Agency staff, management Local government staff/ management	0.2 equivalent full time	Local government, for example
Workforce development Staff training on active transport (benefits for health, environment, productivity)	Staff delivering the program Management			
Resources Identification of opportunities for pooling resources				

continued

251

continued

Health promotion interventions and capacity-building strategies	Estimated reach	Timelines and by whom	Estimated budget	OPTIONAL Estimated other funding sources
with partner agencies to support the proportion of social marketing strategies and community-based sessions and potential for a peer education program				
Total budget per objective = Total budget per program goal =				

Garrard et al. 2004. Reprinted with kind permission of the Victorian Government, Melbourne

Stage 5: Evaluation

Evaluation involves a systematic assessment of the degree to which an intervention is meeting its objectives. If the budget allows, this should first be carried out early in a campaign to correct any deficiencies or capitalise on any new opportunities that present themselves, as well as at the end of the program. (For process, impact and outcome evaluation methods, see McKenzie, Neiger & Thackery 2012; Healy & Zimmerman 2009; and Valente 2002.)

In general, evaluation measures should be developed and in place before a program is initiated. However, in some circumstances, changes in events as a result of the intervention may lead to a modification of the program.

Funding for evaluation is often not included in budgets allocated by those not appreciating the importance of evaluation. However, it is often these same funding sources (e.g. community leaders, politicians) who use evaluation results to either confirm or deny the value of their funding allocations when these are put under scrutiny. Funding for evaluation should be seen as an integral part of any health promotion program. A 'rule of thumb' for this allocation would be approximately 10 per cent of the total health promotion budget.

Summary of tasks in stage 5

Main tasks

- Conduct baseline, early stage and end-of-campaign evaluations.
- Measure process objectives (e.g. increases in awareness and knowledge, receipt of messages, involvement in appropriate actions, improved skills, environmental change).
- Measure outcomes (e.g. using existing databases or carrying out pre- and post-test sampling of BMI, waist circumference).
- Statistical analysis of results.
- Write reports.

Summary

Planning and designing health promotion interventions follow a logical commonsense sequence. Regardless of terminology in the different models, and regardless of whether it is a limited duration campaign or a long-term program being planned, most approaches begin with some sort of problem identification, then move to a selection of goals, followed by identification and consideration of alternative strategies to achieve those goals, testing and refinement of the strategies before full implementation, monitoring the implementation and using that information to further refine or revise the program components, and ongoing evaluation of outcomes.

Donovan and Henley (2010) note that a key point to remember is that subsequent stages can only be as good as the preceding stages, and the needs-assessment/problem-identification stage is the most important of all. Another key point is that the process is iterative and recursive, with later stages informing earlier stages, especially when pre-testing of methods and materials begins.

Finally, no health promotion is immune from commercial or political interference. Where possible, therefore, program planning should include contingency components to respond to these.

References

Batini, C., & Donovan, R.J., 2001, *Drinking and Driving in the Great Southern: Perceptions of Practices, Priorities and Preventives*, Stage One Qualitative Research Report to Great Southern Public Health Services, NFO Donovan Research, Perth, Western Australia.

Campbell, M.K., Demark-Wahnefried, W., Symons, M., Kalzbeek, W.D., Dodds, J., Cowan, A., Jackson, B., Motsinger, B., Hoben, K., Lashley, J., Demissie, S.,

& McClelland, J.W., 1999, Fruit and vegetable consumption and prevention of cancer: The Black Churches United for Better Health Project *Am J Public Health* 89(9):1390–6.

Cox, CC., 2003, *ACSMs Worksite Health Promotion Manual: A Guide to Building and Sustaining Healthy Worksites*, Human Kinetics, Illinois.

Donovan, R.J., & Henley, N., 2010, *Social Marketing: An International Perspective,* Cambridge University Press, Cambridge.

Edelman, C., Mandel, C.L., & Edelman C.L., 2002, *Health Promotion Throughout the Lifespan* (5th edn), Mosby, St Louis, Missouri.

Garrard, J., Lewis, B. Keleher, H., Tunny, N., Burke L., Harper S., & Round R., 2004, *Planning for Healthy Communities: Reducing the Risk of Cardiovascular Disease through Healthier Environments and Lifestyles,* Victorian Government Department of Human Services, Melbourne.

Green L.W., & Kreuter, M., 1999, *Health Promotion Planning: An Educational and Ecological Approach* (3rd edn), McGraw Hill, New York.

Green, L.W., & Kreuter, M.W., 2005, *Health Promotion Planning: An Educational and Ecological Approach* (4th edn), McGraw-Hill, New York.

Healy, B.J., & Zimmerman, R.S., 2009, *The New World of Health Promotion: New Program Development, Implementation and Evaluation,* Jones and Bartlett, Sudbury, Massachusetts.

Jones, S.C., & Donovan, R.J., 2004, Does theory inform practice in health promotion in Australia? *Health Educ Res* 19(1):1–14.

McKenzie, J.F., Neiger, B.L., & Thackery, R., 2012, *Planning, Implementing and Evaluating Health Promotion Programs: A Primer* (6th edn), Jones and Bartlett, Sudbury, Massachusets.

Murray, R.B., & Zentner, J.P., 2001, *Health Promotion Strategies Through the Life Span* (7th edn), Prentice Hall, New Jersey.

Ransdell, L., 2001, Using the PRECEDE–PROCEED model to increase productivity in health education faculty, *Int J Health Educ* 4(1):276–82.

Spark, R., 1999, *Developing Health Promotion Methods in Remote Aboriginal Communities,* Unpublished doctoral dissertation, Curtin University, Perth, Western Australia.

Valente T.W., 2002, *Evaluating Health Promotion Programs,* Oxford University Press, New York.

Viola, A., 2002, *Building Healthy Queensland Communities Inaugural Seminar,* Health Promotion Queensland, Brisbane.

Woolf, S.H., Jonas, S., & Lawrence, R.S., 1996, *Health Promotion and Disease Prevention in Clinical Practice.* Lippincott, Williams & Wilkins, Philadelphia, P.A.

Wright, A., McGorry, P.D., Harris, M.G., Jorm, A.F., & Pennell, K., 2006, Development and evaluation of a youth mental health community awareness campaign—The Compass Strategy, *BMC Public Health* 6(215):1–9.

chapter 11

Skills, tools and competencies for health promotion

Summary of main points

- *Skills* are defined as the ability to successfully facilitate a particular process. *Tools* are a means of doing this through available techniques.
- Health promotion practitioners need skills and tools that cross the boundaries of many other professions.
- The wider the health promotion practitioner's repertoire of skills, the greater the options available for dealing with any issue.
- While *content* knowledge is important, *process* skills differentiate the health promotion practitioner from other health professionals.
- Skills range from writing, community facilitation, advocacy and political acumen to clinical, evaluation and social marketing ability.
- The competencies required for health promotion have been specified in professional standards documents.

The need for specialist skills

As an art/science, health promotion requires a unique combination of skills and operational tools that cross the boundaries of several other professions. At one extreme, there are advantages in having clinical skills for dealing with patients/clients on a one-to-one basis, whether as a medical practitioner or as an allied health professional. At the other extreme, there are political, lobbying and social advocacy skills that can help set the agenda for changes at the population level. Within each of these areas there are established tools such as clinical methods, communication skills, screening tests and educational approaches for enabling the process of health promotion to occur. Not all may be within the repertoire of a single health promotion practitioner. However, the wider the practitioner's repertoire, the greater the options available for dealing with any particular issue. Developing applied skills and ability to use tools also widens the opportunity for employment for health promotion practitioners outside the health sector, such as in community development, advertising, market research, media, journalism or public policy.

In contrast to the 'content' of health issues, which involves some basic biological, psychological and epidemiological knowledge, skills and tools facilitate the 'process' of health promotion. As with this text in general, some level of health science content is assumed. A range of process skills for disseminating this content and implementing health promotion initiatives for an intended audience is outlined below. This is not definitive and new skills will need to be added as new knowledge and new tools become available. Skills are defined as *the ability to successfully facilitate a particular process.* Tools are *a means of doing this through available techniques.* It is these that differentiate the health promotion practitioner from other health professionals. In the final part of this chapter we list a number of competencies regarded as desirable for health promotion practitioners under the stage headings described in the SOPIE model described in Chapter 10.

Skills for health promoters

The following is a list of essential skills for health promotion professionals.

- *Organisational and planning ability*—any health promotion intervention requires detailed organisation and planning and the ability to work in concert with locally identified personnel.
- *Interviewing and listening skills*—formative work in the early stages of any project requires the ability to interview key stakeholders and translate this information into functional interventions. An ability to develop empathy and communicate with a variety of different groups that may include Indigenous, minority and culturally and linguistically diverse (CALD) groups are also vital.
- *Teaching ability*—this is required at different levels to increase knowledge among professionals, stakeholders and community members and may include didactic lecturing, interactive learning processes or education through a range of different communication methods.
- *Group facilitation*—the ability to organise and run small groups and understand group dynamics is essential for a number of processes in health promotion, including those listed above.
- *Media skills*—the basics of transmitting health messages through the select use of appropriate media channels. The ability to use mass and limited-reach media is a valuable skill for successful health promotion.

- *Ability to work collaboratively with a range of different disciplines*—including developing and implementing specific program components. This includes the ability to interact with a range of other skilled personnel, such as graphic artists and creative personnel, statisticians and demographers, medical and health professionals, social and community welfare professionals, and academics and researchers.
- *Report-writing ability*—writing at the academic level is necessary to pass on information about successes and failures achieved within any program. All interventions should be conducted with a view to potential publication (including in journals such as the *Health Promotion Journal of Australia*, the *Australian and New Zealand Journal of Public Health*, etc.). This includes the ability to successfully 'translate' scientific evidence into understandable language.
- *Evaluation skills*—the ability to evaluate a project at any of a number of levels (process, impact and outcome) is vital to improve future interventions (and to receive ongoing support for health promotion).
- *Political skills*—'political' is meant here in the broad sense of understanding interactions between professionals, stakeholders and the community in general, particularly where these interactions may be able to influence healthy public policy.
- *Ability to source and understand evidence-based content material*—although not everything about a health issue needs to be understood to communicate the key aspects, it is important for health promotion professionals to know how to access the scientific literature to confirm areas of possible controversy and understand the evidence base. This involves skills in internet searching techniques and an understanding of levels of acceptance of scientific evidence.

Additional desirable skills include:

- *Ability to facilitate community development/organisational processes*—the process of working in different sized communities and enabling these to develop mechanisms for health promotion from within is a vital component of many health promotion interventions.
- *Clinical (one-to-one) counselling*—this represent the 'grassroots' of health promotion that is often overlooked by many non-clinical professionals. However, it is a useful skill for anyone likely to be involved in facilitating behaviour change, providing the practitioner is appropriately clinically qualified or even registered to deliver the health information.
- *Social marketing skills*—given the widespread adoption of commercial marketing techniques in health promotion interventions, an understanding of the disciplines of marketing and consumer behaviour would assist health promotion practitioners working with professionals in these areas.

- *Survey and sampling knowledge*—although health promotion professionals themselves may not require this, an awareness of the appropriate techniques enables a more effective supervision of planning and evaluation research.
- *'Train the trainer' skills*—much health promotion involves working directly with health professionals to expand content knowledge in areas such as infectious diseases, physical fitness, nutrition, weight control, stress management and drug abuse. The ability to build capacity through trainer training is a useful skill.

CASE STUDY **11.1**

Some general principles for working in different cultural settings, including developing countries

There a number of principles involved in health promotion activities that, although often not defined, are worthy of consideration, particularly in cultural sub-groups and in developing countries. The list outlined below has been developed from personal experience of the authors in this capacity.

- *Things do not happen quickly*—health behaviour change can be a slow process in any culture or community. Many interventions first require awareness, then agreement, then consensus of the key stakeholders involved before any health-promoting activities take place.
- *Plan ahead*—time is always best spent in a country or community when visits are well planned in advance.
- *Find a local advocate or collaborator to manage the process*—success will depend on one or a small number of enthusiastic advocates who can help drive the program from within. Such individuals may or may not necessarily come from the health sector, but should be respected in the community. They should be used as a vital resource and provided with relevant information/training.
- *Devolve 'ownership' of the program to the community*—any program will be more likely to be successful if people in the home community drive it on an ongoing basis. Long-term health change requires continuous input and outside assistants cannot and should not be expected to provide this on an ongoing basis. The program must belong to the community with the practitioner or consultant merely acting as a catalyst.
- *Expect 'down' times*—these are inevitable and may result from changes in plans or failure of meetings to materialise to whole visits that may be less productive than initially planned. Weather (particularly during monsoon seasons) is sometimes a limiting factor in tropical countries in the Asia–Pacific region, and this may be a consideration in planning short-term projects.

- *Appreciate the culture*—first visits to a new community or country will always involve a 'fast learning curve' when it is necessary to learn cultural practices and mores. This should involve familiarisation with the community and its culture beforehand.
- *Develop rapport*—as with any one-to-one clinical relationship, no behaviour or local policy change is likely to occur until trust and rapport is developed with the client (in this case the community). This will take time and hence the early stages of any program should be spent nurturing this relationship with all aspects of the population (e.g. local media, stakeholders, health sector personnel).
- *Work within the existing frameworks and systems*—as early as possible in a program, time should be spent in consultation with those in the local health and other related services who are likely to have significant influence. This is often not just the local doctors, but nurses, allied health and other health workers, recreational officers and even traditional healers in a village context.
- *Work with, not against, local structures*—religion forms a large part of life in many developing countries, but in some cases (e.g. the Pacific) it can play an unwitting role in the facilitation of certain (potentially unhealthy) practices such as feasting and inactivity. On the other hand, church leaders can be major instigators of change if they become part of the solution to the health problems these practices can create for their communities. Church leaders can also become key advocates for health promotion.
- *Don't assume that what works in one country or community will work in another*—while learnings are often transferable, a basic principle in designing health promotion interventions is the three words *'it all depends'*. This means that interventions—and their implementation in particular—must be specific to the culture or place.
- *Know your boundaries*—most cultures have multiple layers, some of which may be revealed to the short-term visitor, but others that are less obvious and even undisclosed. It is not only a mistake to think that this can be accessed by an outsider, but could also be offensive. Hence, while you may be invited to participate in certain activities in a community, do not assume you are invited to other activities.
- *As far as possible, check your opinions with others before making conclusions*—working in different cultures often means coming to conclusions based on one's own culture. By working with others in the same field, ideas can be compared and conclusions checked before basing further actions on what could be a misconception.
- *Begin with humility*—an outsider can find his or her input blocked by locals or other consultants who may feel threatened by an over-assertive insensitive approach. Until rapport is established, humility is imperative, combined with polite listening and questioning skills.
- *Always ask beforehand if something can be done, and how*—with tasks such as filming, conducting training, meeting stakeholders and so on, it is important to

continued

259

continued

find out if what you want to do is acceptable in that context. In some instances, status may prohibit the use of certain protocols, and ignoring this may mean permanent difficulty in further operations. A trusted advocate can advise on the appropriate behaviours.

- *Build local capacity*—avoid being a 'parachute consultant' by maintaining relationships and support in the period following your visit (particularly if this is a short-term project).
- *Carry out everything with a view to documentation for sustainability*—while not all health promotion activities are publishable, it is important to keep scientific publication in mind as an end process of any potential action, providing locals are involved or acknowledged and drafts are approved by local stakeholders. Too often, health promotion interventions, both successful and unsuccessful, are not reported in the literature, leaving future projects to 're-invent the wheel'.

Egger 2004; see also Demaio 2008 for the WHO's
eight principles of Culturally Appropriate Health Promotion

Competencies required of the health promotion professional

Below we list the main competencies considered essential or desirable for health promotion professionals in Australia. This has been adapted from a review of competencies initially completed in 1994 and since updated in 2003 and 2008 (Shilton et al. 2003, 2008). The use of these competencies has been mapped against international benchmarks to advance professional standards in general and for advocacy to ensure health promotion is better resourced and prioritised by policy makers globally (Shilton 2009). Health promotion competencies are listed below under the stage headings provided in the SOPIE model discussed in Chapter 10.

Situational analysis

Competencies include being able to:

1. identify behavioural, environmental and organisational factors that promote or compromise health
2. assist and involve communities in identifying needs and setting priorities for health promotion
3. identify and source data on health needs
4. critically analyse relevant literature.

Objective setting

Competencies include being able to:

1. formulate appropriate and measurable objectives
2. develop logical, sequenced and sustainable programs based on theory and evidence
3. communicate verbally and listen reflectively
4. debate health-related issues using evidence-based arguments
5. consider and apply theory to health promotion planning, implementation and research.

Planning

Competencies include be able to:

1. establish appropriate partnerships and facilitate collaborative action
2. involve community members and stakeholders in program planning and action
3. apply a range of approaches to health education
4. coordinate production of appropriate program support materials
5. liaise and collaborate with other professionals and organisations
6. use technology-based systems and resources such as the internet.

Implementation

Competencies include being able to:

1. assist, support and build capacity in service providers and clinical workers
2. apply interpersonal skills (e.g. negotiation, team work, motivation, conflict resolution, decision making, problem solving)
3. apply mass media, group, healthy policy and structural/environmental strategies
4. write and apply interviewee skills for media
5. be able to articulate health promotion jargon into salient language
6. devolve programs to the community
7. work as part of a team.

Evaluation

Competencies include being able to:

1. identify appropriate evaluation designs
2. interpret and communicate evaluation findings
3. monitor programs and adjust objectives.

A final look—health promotion: the human factor

Together with the strategies and methods discussed in this book, the skills and competencies discussed in this chapter help to define some of the requirements of a successful health promotion practitioner. They, along with relevant academic training and professional development and networking (see Case study 11.2 on the Australian Health Promotion Association), provide a useful template for contemporary health promotion practice. However, no program should ever underestimate the power of the human factor: the *person* making it happen. For that reason the passionate health promotion practitioner requires not just personal and process skills and academic training, but a more than adequate supply of 'fire in the belly'—a belief in and commitment to the value of health promotion in contributing to improvements in human health—as well as improvements in the less specific, but equally important area of quality of life.

CASE STUDY **11.2**

Professional developing and networking—the Australian Health Promotion Association

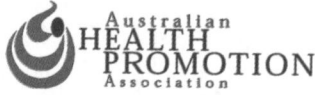

From humble beginnings in Western Australia in 1985, the Australian Health Promotion Association (AHPA) now has a large and diverse membership with branches in all Australian states and the Northern Territory. AHPA's overall goal is to encourage and support best practice in health promotion so that everyone can enjoy good health. AHPA's vision, mission and value statements are shown below. With a respected professional journal, the *Health Promotion Journal of Australia*, an annual national conference and numerous professional development opportunities, membership of AHPA provides excellent professional networking, particularly for new health promotion practitioners or those working in professional or geographic isolation. (See www.healthpromotion.org.au.)

Vision

AHPA acknowledged as a national voice for health promotion in Australia and a major contributor to the health of all Australians.

Mission

To advocate for health promotion, the health promotion workforce, and best health promotion practice.

Values

AHPA's values are those enshrined in the Ottawa Charter for Health Promotion. They include equity, social justice, and shared responsibility for health. AHPA's values are expressed in professional excellence, and ethical practice.

References

Demaio, A., 2008, *Local Wisdom and Health Promotion: Barrier or Catalyst*, WHO, Geneva.

Egger, G., 2004, Health promotion consultant's instructional manual, unpublished WHO report.

Shilton, T., 2009, Health promotion competencies: providing a road map for health promotion to assume a prominent role in global health, *Global Health Promot* 16(2):42–6.

Shilton, T., Howat, P., James, R., Hutchins, C., & Burke, L., 2008, Potential uses of health promotion competencies, *Health Promot J Aust* 19(3):184–8.

Shilton T., Howat P., James R., & Lower T., 2003, Review of competencies for Australian health promotion, *IUHPE Promot Educ* 10(4):162–70.

Index